WELLES-TURNER MEMORIAL LIBRARY
GLASTONBURY, CT 06033

Spaced Retrieval
Step by Step

DISCARDED BY
WELLES-TURNER
MEMORIAL LIBRARY
GLASTONBURY, CT

D1597335

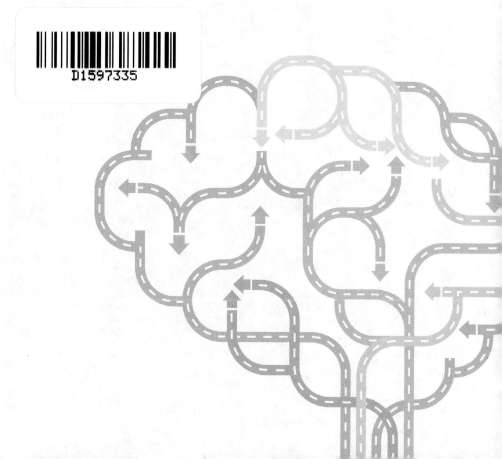

WELLES-TURNER MEMORIAL LIBRARY
GLASTONBURY, CT 06033

DISCARDED
WELLES-TUR...
MEMORIAL LIB...RY
GLASTONBURY, CT

Spaced Retrieval Step by Step

AN EVIDENCE-BASED MEMORY INTERVENTION

by
Jeanette E. Benigas, Ph.D., CCC-SLP
Jennifer A. Brush, M.A., CCC-SLP
Gail M. Elliot, B.A.Sc., M.A.

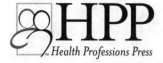
HPP
Health Professions Press

Baltimore • London • Sydney

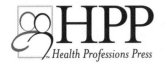

Health Professions Press, Inc.
Post Office Box 10624
Baltimore, Maryland 21285-0624

www.healthpropress.com

Copyright © 2016 by Health Professions Press, Inc.
All rights reserved.

Interior and cover designs by Mindy Dunn.
Typeset by Mindy Dunn.
Manufactured in the United States of America by Versa Press, East Peoria, Illinois.

The information provided in this book is in no way meant to substitute for the advice or opinion of a medical, legal, or other professional or expert. This book is sold without warranties of any kind, express or implied, and the publisher and author disclaim any liability, loss, or damage caused by the contents of this book.

Professional and family care partners who purchase *Spaced Retrieval Step by Step: An Evidence-Based Memory Intervention* are granted permission to print or photocopy the downloadable resources from the HPP website for their own use in caregiving. Please be sure the credit line to the book appears on each copy you make. The downloadable resources comprise PDF files. None of the materials may be reproduced to generate revenue for any program or individual. Unauthorized use is prosecutable under federal law.

Library of Congress Cataloging-in-Publication Data

Names: Benigas, Jeanette E., author. | Brush, Jennifer A., author. | Elliot,
   Gail M., 1957– , author.
Title: Spaced retrieval step by step : an evidence-based memory intervention
   / by Jeanette E. Benigas, Jennifer A. Brush, Gail M. Elliot.
Description: Baltimore, Maryland : Health Professions Press, Inc., [2016] |
   Includes bibliographical references.
Identifiers: LCCN 2015043690 (print) | LCCN 2015044822 (ebook) | ISBN
   9781938870460 (pbk.) | ISBN 9781938870569 (ebook) | ISBN 9781938870569
   (epub)
Subjects: | MESH: Memory Disorders—rehabilitation. |
   Dementia—rehabilitation. | Mental Recall. | Rehabilitation—methods. |
   Time Factors.
Classification: LCC RC394.M46 (print) | LCC RC394.M46 (ebook) | NLM WM 173.7
   | DDC 616.8/3--dc23
LC record available at http://lccn.loc.gov/2015043690

British Library Cataloguing-in-Publication data are available from the British Library.

This book is dedicated to
all of the people living with memory loss
as well as their care partners.

Contents

Downloadable Resources

DOWNLOAD

The following resources are available for download at www.healthpropress.com/benigas-downloads (use password [case sensitive]: SjnE3Nxq).

Professional and family care partners who purchase *Spaced Retrieval Step by Step: An Evidence-Based Memory Intervention* are granted permission to print or photocopy the downloadable resources from the HPP website for their own use in caregiving. Please be sure the credit line to the book appears on each copy you make. The downloadable resources comprise PDF files. None of the materials may be reproduced to generate revenue for any program or individual. Unauthorized use is prosecutable under federal law.

About the Authors

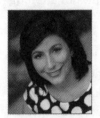 **Jeanette E. Benigas, Ph.D., CCC-SLP,** is an Assistant Professor of Communication Sciences and Disorders at West Chester University (PA). Her extensive clinical experience as a speech-language pathologist has included work in pediatrics in both private practice and school settings as well as with adults in post-acute, long-term care, and home health settings. Dr. Benigas's research interests include improving quality of life for persons with dementia, specifically those who have difficulties eating and swallowing. Her research has incorporated the use of Spaced Retrieval to teach swallowing strategies to avoid unwanted dietary modifications. She has traveled nationally to speak with other SLPs and continues to practice privately. Dr. Benigas received a Master's in Speech-Language Pathology from Eastern Michigan University and a Doctorate in Speech and Hearing Science with an Interdisciplinary Specialization in Aging from The Ohio State University.

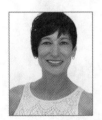 **Jennifer A. Brush, M.A., CCC-SLP,** understands the particular needs of healthcare organizations and families who are engaged in dementia care and has more than 20 years of experience as both a leading researcher and direct-care coach in this complex field. She is an international speaker and recognized speech-language pathologist known for her work in the areas of memory, swallowing, and environmental interventions for people with dementia. Brush has served as the Principal Investigator on applied research grants that have examined issues pertaining to HIV/AIDS, dementia, hearing impairment, dining, dysphagia, and the long-term care environment. Her research and consulting in the area of environmental modifications has resulted in improved functioning for people with dementia. Brush is the co-author of several books: *Creative Connections in Dementia Care: Engaging Activities to Enhance Communication; I Care: A Handbook for Care Partners of People with Dementia; Environment & Communication Assessment Toolkit for Dementia Care (ECAT);* and *A Therapy Technique for Improving Memory: Spaced Retrieval.* Learn more at www.BrushDevelopment.com.

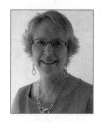 **Gail M. Elliot, B.A.Sc., M.A.,** a gerontologist and dementia specialist, is the Founder and CEO of DementiAbility Enterprises, Inc. In 2012, Elliot retired from her position as Assistant Director at Gilbrea Centre for Studies in Aging at McMaster University to pursue her lifelong goal of changing the face of dementia by helping those with the disease live to their full potential. She is passionate about creating a better world for those who need a voice and support. Resources and strategies developed by Elliot have been implemented across Canada as well as internationally. Elliot's DementiAbility and Communication courses are part of McMaster University's Geriatric Certificate Program. She works closely with the Occupational Therapists Association of Hong Kong, Montessori Australia Foundation, and colleagues in the United States. Elliot is the author of the book *Montessori Methods for Dementia™: Focusing on the Person in the Prepared Environment; Memory Aids for Dementia;* and *Helping Me . . . Helping You: Practical Approaches for Caregivers.* She is co-author of *Checklist for Change: A Guide for Facilitating Culture Change in Long-Term Care.* She is also editor of several titles available as part of the series *Carry on Reading in Dementia.* Learn more at www.DementiAbility.com.

Acknowledgments

I would like to thank my husband Jonathan W. Hunt for his unending love, support, and grace through this project. His encouragement made the hard work a little bit easier and I am blessed to have him in my corner every day.

—*Jeanette Benigas*

The authors wish to personally thank the following individuals: our colleagues Michelle Bourgeois, Ph.D., CCC-SLP, Renee Kinder, M.S., CCC-SLP, and Pamela Smith, Ph.D., CCC-SLP; West Chester University students Chelsea Bauder, Zach Davis, Siobhan Groves, Chelsea Linton, and Megan Simmons; and everyone on the Health Professions Press team who made this project not only possible, but something to be proud of: Julie Chávez, Cecilia González, Kimberly Beauchamp, Kaitlin Konecke, Mindy Dunn, and Mary Magnus. Without all of their contributions and support, this book would not have been written.

Preface

In 1996, I (Jennifer Brush) was working at a long-term care community. I spent the majority of my time on the memory care units helping people with dementia lead more independent lives. While working there, I learned about Spaced Retrieval and began implementing this memory-training strategy with people who had Alzheimer's disease, Parkinson's disease, traumatic brain injury, aphasia, and other conditions that cause memory loss. I was amazed that with practice verbalizing information, my clients were able to remember the material over increasing amounts of time. These people each faced challenges related to memory loss, yet they were remembering important facts, names, and tasks that were a part of their daily lives.

With great enthusiasm, I taught this strategy to the occupational therapists, physical therapists, and other speech-language pathologists with whom I worked. We then began teaching residents to remember essential information, including how to use their walkers, lock their wheelchair brakes, find their rooms, and use swallowing strategies. We were excited to have had so much success in helping them lead more independent lives. I went on to co-author a book on the approach titled *A Therapy Technique for Improving Memory: Spaced Retrieval* (Brush & Camp, 1998), and have used Spaced Retrieval with countless individuals living with memory loss. Many other clinicians and researchers around the world have also successfully implemented the strategy through their work.

In publishing *Spaced Retrieval Step by Step: An Evidence-Based Memory Intervention,* my two co-authors and I are sharing new tips, current research, and fresh ideas for how Spaced Retrieval can be used to teach people with dementia and other forms of memory loss to better recall important information. I feel fortunate to have written this book with two friends and colleagues who have used Spaced Retrieval in the home, hospital, long-term care, and rehabilitation settings. Jeanette Benigas, Assistant Professor of Communication Sciences and Disorders at West Chester University, completed her doctoral dissertation in Spaced Retrieval and travels nationally to teach the strategy to other speech-language pathologists. Gail Elliot, a gerontologist, teaches this intervention to families and healthcare professionals throughout Canada as well as many other parts of the world.

We hope that our efforts will inspire you to include this easy intervention as part of your daily practice in helping to restore a greater level of independence and self-efficacy for people living with memory loss.

Jennifer A. Brush, M.A., CCC-SLP

Introduction

Spaced Retrieval (SR) is a memory-training strategy that is used to teach people with memory loss new or previously known information. The objective of SR is to help people with cognitive impairment store information in their long-term memory so that they can better recall important details, such as when to take medications or how to use a walker. This objective is achieved by working with the person to practice remembering information until the information can be easily accessed and retrieved when needed. SR emphasizes setting the person up for success by beginning with short time intervals between practices and then systematically increasing the time between each practice as the person successfully recalls the details he or she needs to remember. The success of SR is based on exposure to, and practice of, specific information. It is both the exposure and the practice that increase the probability of remembering. The best part about SR is that any care partner can use this strategy. Care partners can be family members, speech-language pathologists, physical therapists, occupational therapists, nurses, social workers, and home health aides. The fact that a wide range of people can use this multidisciplinary approach contributes to its effectiveness. This book is meant to be accessible to all care partners—family, healthcare professionals, and friends.

Why Is Spaced Retrieval Important?

According to global estimates, 47.5 million people are living with dementia (World Health Organization [WHO], 2015). The statistics are expected to double every 20 years to 66 million by 2030 and to 115 million by 2050 (Alzheimer's Disease International, 2013). Dementia has been referred to as a worldwide epidemic.

Currently, there is no cure for dementia. As researchers continue to search for a cure and develop pharmacological treatments to lessen the impact of dementia-related symptoms, care partners need to put evidence-based interventions into practice now to ease the challenges that are confronting people with memory loss conditions. Care partners have used SR to eliminate repetitive questioning, reduce anxiety, improve recall of important facts, and increase safety for people with memory loss of varying causes. SR has proven effective as a behavioral treatment for improved independence, safety, and quality of life by enhancing recall of functional information to successfully complete tasks. Spaced Retrieval has also become a leading intervention by improving cognitive-linguistic function for individuals with memory loss. The American Speech-Language-Hearing Association (ASHA) has recognized SR as an evidence-based practice for people with mild to severe cognitive-communicative impairments (ASHA, 2012). Although SR methodologies are variable, research has found that SR can help improve the acquisition, retention, and generalization of trained information and skills. These improvements can be retained for up to several months following the completion of training (Hopper et al., 2005; Hopper et al., 2013).

How Can This Book Help?

Unfortunately, many care partners often focus on the losses and disability related to dementia rather than on the abilities that are spared and that can still be enhanced. Many people assume that people with memory and cognitive impairments cannot succeed in learning new or previously known information. If care partners know how to support and enhance memory by helping the person to remember needed information, however, the person can experience successful outcomes rather than live with continual challenges and frustrations that affect his or her safety and self-esteem. By building on a person's abilities, we can compensate for the deficits associated with memory and cognitive loss.

The authors, as well as clinicians and numerous researchers, have used SR successfully with many people, including those with Alzheimer's disease, Parkinson's disease, traumatic brain injury, aphasia, and other conditions that cause memory loss. We are excited to bring this life-changing strategy to you. Our hope is that this book will allow you to implement SR successfully as a care partner and that this intervention will enhance the memory, well-being, safety, and independence of those in your care who are living with memory loss.

About the Book

Several features in this book are designed to assist the reader. At the end of this Introduction is a useful Glossary of Terms. Throughout the book, icons are used to call attention to topic categories so the reader can quickly locate examples of how to implement the strategy for a specific need. The topic categories are defined in an Icon Key that follows the Glossary of Terms. Preceding Chapter 1 is an engaging timeline of the published research on SR. Helpful case studies are interwoven throughout the book to demonstrate real-world examples of SR in action and provide the reader with a practical model to follow. Finally, Chapters 2 and 3 include sample forms that are discussed in the text. The forms are suitable for copying for ease of use and are also available for download as PDF files by logging on to www.healthpropress.com/benigas-downloads (use password [case sensitive]: SjnE3Nxq).

Readers of this book will find step-by-step guidance on how to use SR procedures to increase safety, support independence, and enhance cognitive-linguistic function for any person who struggles to remember. Chapter 1 discusses the theoretical foundation of memory and why SR works. In Chapter 2, we provide practical approaches for care partners with an emphasis on helping them to put SR into practice. The reader will learn how to identify the person's needs and desires, create the SR format of *lead question* and *response* that will support and address the person's needs, implement the protocol for SR practice, and make modifications to increase success. Chapter 3 introduces tools to support SR practice, including physical supports, such as continuous visual cues and external memory aids, as well as social and environmental supports. Chapter 4 presents practical case examples that illustrate how to implement and personalize SR for a variety of individuals. Finally, Chapter 5 provides a chronological summary of many published studies related to SR. This comprehensive outline of research illustrates the breadth and depth of the evidence in support of the SR strategy.

Glossary of Terms

Booster Sessions: Additional SR practices used after the initial SR training has been discontinued. Booster sessions can be helpful for long-term retention if the information continues to be important for the individual.

Care Partner: A professional, family member, friend, or other individual who shares in planning and implementing care with, and for, a person living with memory loss.

Continuous Visual Cue: Involves placing the response to the lead question in writing in the person's line of sight during each SR practice, which reinforces both learning and retention.

Errorless Learning: Contributes to the likelihood of increased long-term retention and supports learning the correct response by eliminating errors as well as the process of searching to find the response during the SR practice.

Lead Question: The prompt or cue in the form of a question that elicits the response.

Need or Desire: The first step when preparing to implement SR is to identify the person's need or desire. A need is something that is very important; it is necessary or required. A desire is a wish or a want.

Practice: The opportunity for the care partner to present the lead question and for the person with memory loss to provide the response.

Response: The piece of information and/or physical task that will help the person meet the identified need or desire.

Spacing Effect: The spacing effect is based on the finding that information is learned and retrieved more effectively when practices are spaced over time. SR was designed around the spacing effect by having the care partner create successive practices at increasing time intervals.

Time Interval: The deliberate amount of seconds or minutes used in between each SR practice. The time interval should begin after the response is given or the physical task is performed.

Spaced Retrieval Icon Key

 Safety

 Activities of Daily Living and Independence

 Orientation and Wayfinding

 Name Recognition

 Details and Information

 Spaced Retrieval

 Spacing Effect

 Errorless Learning

 Remember Things to Do

 Names of Objects

 Eating or Swallowing Behaviors

 Social Skills

 Literature Review

Spaced Retrieval Research Timeline

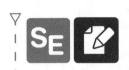

Ebbinghaus, 1885/1913
This study laid the foundation for SR. The subject learned nonsense syllables by memorization and then was later tested for free recall.

Spitzer, 1939
Expanded retrieval was used to examine the rate of forgetting in comparison to subject ability.

Peterson et al., 1963
The spacing effect was used to train subjects to recall pairs of words and numbers.

Hogan & Kintsch, 1971
The spacing effect was used to train subjects to recall word lists.

Glenberg, 1977
The spacing effect was used to train subjects to recall word lists.

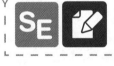

Landauer & Bjork, 1978
The spacing effect was used to teach subjects first and last names.

Hello
Eleanor

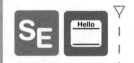

Glenberg, 1979
The spacing effect was used to train subjects to recall word pairs.

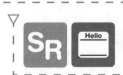

Schater et al., 1985
SR was used to train subjects to recall faces in correspondence to names, hometowns, and hobbies.

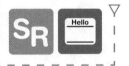

Camp, 1989
SR was used to train subjects to recall face–name associations.

Balota et al., 1989
The spacing effect was used to show that older adults performed worse than younger adults in recalling information.

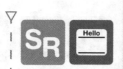

Camp & Schaller, 1989
SR was used to teach one subject the name of a care partner.

McKitrick et al., 1992
SR was used to train subjects to recall tasks for future actions.

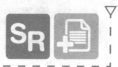

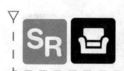

Abrahams & Camp, 1993
SR was used to train two subjects to recall target objects from the Boston Naming Test.

McKitrick & Camp, 1993
SR was used to train subjects to recall familiar objects from the Boston Naming Test.

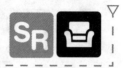

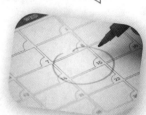

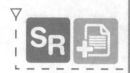

Stevens et al., 1993
SR was used to teach one subject to use a calendar to perform weekly tasks.

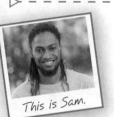

This is Sam.

Wilson et al., 1994
Errorless learning was used to teach subjects the names of people and objects.

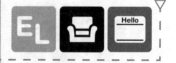

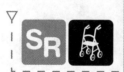

Bird et al., 1995
SR was used to decrease subjects' problem behaviors.

Bird & Kinsella, 1996
SR and a written word cue were used to train subjects to perform motor tasks.

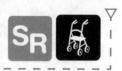

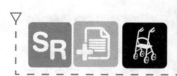

Hayden & Camp, 1996
SR was used to teach subjects with Parkinson's disease a verbal, motor, and motor–verbal task.

Carruth, 1997
SR, combined with singing, was used to train subjects to recall face–name associations.

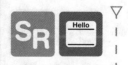

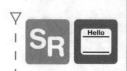

Camp & Foss, 1997
SR was used to teach one subject to recall a care partner's name to reduce behavior perceived as difficult.

Brush & Camp, 1998a
SR was used as a functional tool for helping subjects reach speech-language therapy goals.

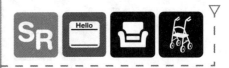

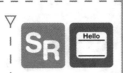

Brush & Camp, 1998b
SR was used to train one subject compensatory strategies for safe swallowing.

Hunkin et al., 1998
Errorless learning was used to teach one subject to perform basic word processing tasks.

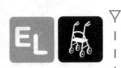

Vanhalle et al., 1998
SR was used to train one subject to recall face–name associations.

Cherry & Simmons-D'Gerolamo, 1999
Subjects learned to recall names of target objects.

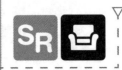

When I eat I:
1. take a small bite
2. chew slowly
3. swallow

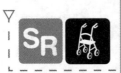

Cherry et al., 1999
SR was used to teach subjects to recall names of everyday objects.

Anderson et al., 2001
SR was used to teach subjects to recall personal information.

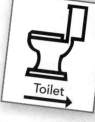

Toilet

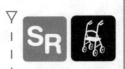

Bird, 2001
SR and a fading cue were used to train subjects to replace undesired behaviors with appropriate ones.

Davis et al., 2001
SR was used to train subjects to improve recall of personal information, face–name associations, and performance on the Verbal Series Attention Test.

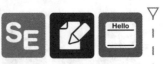

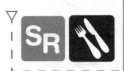

Lee & Camp, 2001
SR was shown to be a useful cognitive intervention for older adults with HIV.

Lekeu et al., 2002
SR was used to train subjects to consult a card posted on the back of a cell phone that had directions for how to use the device.

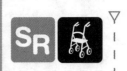

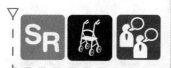

Bourgeois et al., 2003
SR and a modified cuing hierarchy were used to train subjects to enhance social skills, activities of daily living, and participation in activities.

Joltin et al., 2003
SR was used to train subjects to recall over the phone the names of their family members.

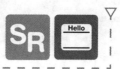

Cherry & Simmons-D'Gerolamo, 2004
SR was used to train subjects to recall names of household objects.

Hawley & Cherry, 2004
SR was used to train subjects to recall names of unfamiliar people.

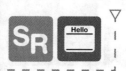

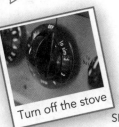

Turn off the stove

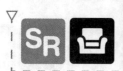

Hochhalter et al., 2004
SR was used to train subjects to recall names of medications.

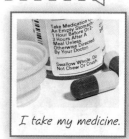

I take my medicine.

Neundorfer et al., 2004
SR was used to train subjects with HIV to improve performance on self-selected functional tasks by using memory aids.

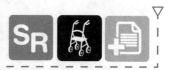

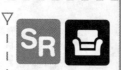

Cherry & Simmons-D'Gerolamo, 2005
SR was used to train subjects to recall everyday objects.

Fridriksson et al., 2005
SR was used to train subjects with aphasia to name objects.

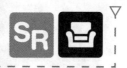

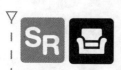

Hochhalter et al., 2005
Two studies were conducted to determine if SR is more effective than other schedules of practice.

Hopper et al., 2005
This systematic review evaluated 15 studies to support the use of SR training for those with dementia.

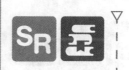

Melton & Bourgeois, 2005
Subjects with brain injury were effectively trained using SR over the telephone.

Turkstra & Bourgeois, 2005
SR and errorless learning were used to train a
person with profound anterograde amnesia to
meet functional memory goals.

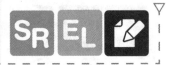

Balota et al., 2006
Various schedules of practice were used to
train subjects to recall word pairs from the
Tulving and Thomas test.

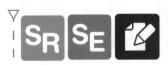

Fridriksson et al., 2006
SR, errorless learning, and massed
practice were used to train subjects
with aphasia to name objects.

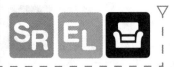

Morrow & Fridriksson, 2006
SR with fixed- and randomized-intervals
was used to train subjects with aphasia
to name target items.

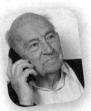

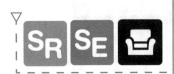

Bourgeois et al., 2007
SR and teaching instruction were used to train
subjects with brain injury over the telephone.

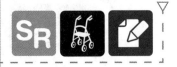

Karpicke & Roediger, 2007a
The spacing effect was used to teach subjects word
lists across multiple study and test trials to examine
the effects of testing on multi-trial free recall.

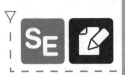

Karpicke & Roediger, 2007b
SR and expanded retrieval were used to teach
subjects vocabulary from the GRE.

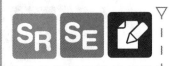

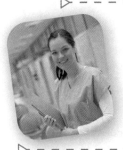

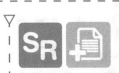

Kinsella et al., 2007
SR was used to train subjects
to perform memory tasks.

Vance & Farr, 2007
The implications for use of SR
by nurses were discussed.

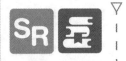

Bishara & Jacoby, 2008
SR and the spacing effect were
used to teach subjects word pairs.

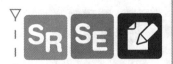

Ellmore et al., 2008
The authors concluded that different amounts
of processing times may be required to retrieve
explicit and implicit memories.

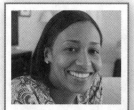

Amy is my day-time nurse

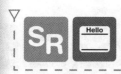

Hawley et al., 2008
SR and expanded retrieval were used to train subjects to recall name–face associations.

Hickey & How, 2008
SR was used to train subjects to read staff nametags to assist with name recollection.

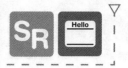

Karpicke & Roediger III, 2008
Effects of repeated studying and testing on learning were examined by teaching subjects a list of foreign language vocabulary words under different conditions.

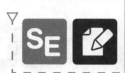

Lee et al., 2008
SR was used to train Korean subjects to recall high imagery words.

Logan & Balota, 2008
SR and expanded retrieval were used with younger and older adults, and both groups experienced substantial benefits, regardless of which form the SR took (expanded or equal interval practice).

Ozgis et al., 2008
SR and standard rehearsal were used to train subjects to perform regular and irregular tasks on a virtual board game.

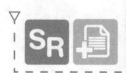

Pavlik & Anderson, 2008
Three learning conditions were used to teach subjects Japanese/English vocabulary words using an algorithm to derive decision criteria for increasing or decreasing spacing.

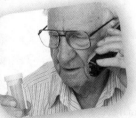

Thivierge et al., 2008
SR and errorless learning were used to train subjects to perform telephone related tasks.

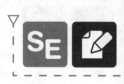

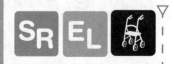

Bier et al., 2009
SR and formal sematic therapy were used to train one subject to name items from pictures.

Cherry et al., 2009
SR was used to train subjects to recall face–name associations. Booster sessions were developed in this study.

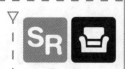

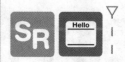

Gonzalez et al., 2009
Errorless learning was used in combination with medication to improve item naming.

Neely et al., 2009
SR was used to examine the effectiveness of a collaborative memory intervention with the subjects and their care partners.

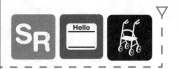

Cherry et al., 2010
SR was used to train subjects to recall name–face–occupation associations.

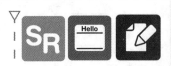

Hopper et al., 2010
The effects of SR on the learning of new and previously known associations were examined.

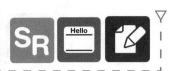

Lin et al., 2010
SR and Montessori-based activities were used to decrease eating difficulties.

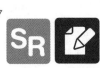

Sumowski et al., 2010
Massed practice, spaced study, and spaced testing were used to train subjects with multiple sclerosis to improve memory performance.

Sumowski et al., 2010
Mass practice, spaced study, and retrieval practice were to observe which procedure is more efficient in improvin memory performance of subjects with brain injury.

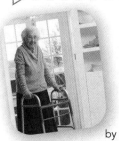

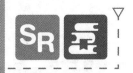

Vance et al., 2010
The implications for use of SR by social workers were discussed.

Haslam et al., 2011
SR and EL were used to train subjects with dementia and brain injury to recall face–name associations.

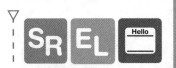

Karpicke & Bauernschmidt, 2011
College students were studied to observe spacing schedules and patterns of response times and the relationship between patterns of response times and final recall.

Karpicke & Blunt, 2011
College students were studied to show that practicing retrieval produces more meaningful learning than elaborative studying with concept mapping.

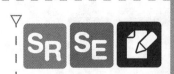

Fiksdal et al., 2012
Memory priming and SR were used to train one subject to recall information from conversations.

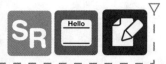

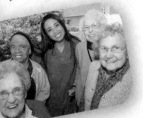

Hunter et al., 2012
SR was used to resolve problem behaviors of subjects in a care facility in Australia. The study also examined how SR can be transferred to staff in an aged care facility once it has been implemented with residents with dementia.

Small, 2012
Three SR conditions were used to train subjects to recall face–name associations, object–word associations, and current events.

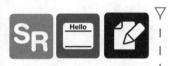

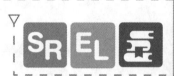

Hopper et al., 2013
Cognitive training in the form of errorless learning and SR was positively reviewed with respect to memory.

Sumowski et al., 2013
Massed restudy, spaced restudy, and SR were used to teach word pairs to subjects with multiple sclerosis.

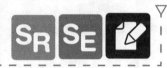

Sam's Chores

Laundry

Take out trash

Sweep leaves off the back deck

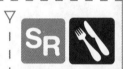

Wu & Lin, 2013
Subjects decreased depressive symptoms and improved nutrition through SR combined with Montessori-based activities.

Han et al., 2014
Subjects learned to recall words derived from the USMART app.

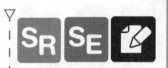

Sumowski et al., 2014
Massed restudy, spaced restudy, and SR were used to teach word pairs to subjects with brain injury.

Coyne et al., 2015
Massed restudy, spaced restudy, and SR were used to teach word pairs to adolescent subjects with brain injury.

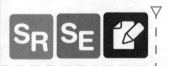

Benigas & Bourgeois, in press
SR and a continuous visual cue were used to teach subjects effective compensatory strategies for swallowing.

The Practice of Spaced Retrieval

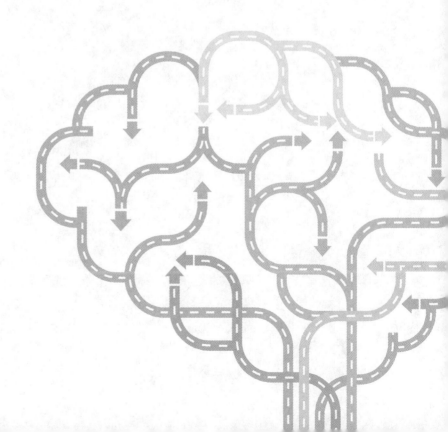

CHAPTER 1

Memory and Spaced Retrieval

This chapter describes the processes involved in memory and discusses the different forms of memory. The chapter also presents Spaced Retrieval (SR) as a strategy for supporting the recall of information and enhancing remaining memory capacity for a person experiencing cognitive loss. Memory involves more than remembering facts and details. Memory is a complex system that involves receiving information, processing the details, manipulating and acting upon the information, and then placing the information into a storage system that can be used when needed at any point in the present or future. Although the extent and location of damage to the brain influence the abilities that remain after the damage has occurred, persons with memory deficits continue to possess a number of strengths and weaknesses associated with learning and retaining information. Each person's ability to learn and remember differs based on the individual, the type of information being processed, and the type of memory loss condition. Because SR is a behavioral intervention that can be used to help people compensate for memory loss, it is helpful to have a basic overview of some of the key elements that are central to understanding our complex memory system.

How Does Memory Work?

In memory, information is gathered through the five senses and is then manipulated, learned, and stored in the brain. The incoming information collected by our senses is first sent to the brain's prefrontal cortex, which is responsible for abstract thinking, regulating behavior, choosing between right and wrong, and predicting the probable outcomes of actions or events. Information is then manipulated through our working memory and short-term memory as it passes through the hippocampus (the area of the brain that forms complex memories), where it is then sent back to the prefrontal cortex for long-term storage. Storage is critical because a person needs to be able to access this information either immediately or later with little effort. Imagine a situation in which you are trying to recall a fact, such as the name of a famous person. When you struggle to remember a fact such as this, you may say, "It's on the tip of my tongue." If someone provides you with a clue, the answer may come immediately. Sometimes we need help retrieving information, and at other times the information comes with no effort.

Accurately recalling information related to trivial questions may not have a serious impact on your day, but the ability to recall certain information is more imperative. For example, an emergency that requires an immediate call for help could be life-threatening if you could not remember that you need to call 911. For information to be accessed with little to no effort, the different components of memory need to work together like the cogs of a gear. When everything works smoothly, we maximize the probability of successfully retrieving key details that we need each minute of the day. The main processing components of memory include encoding (learning), registering, storing, accessing, and retrieving (Baddeley, 1975).

To better understand learning and memory in the brain, consider how a computer operates. Information comes in, is processed, and is placed into an organized file storage system so it can be accessed when needed. If files are not organized in a useful manner, the user cannot easily find the information being sought. Also, if the hard drive is damaged, the user will not be able to gain access to the stored information regardless of how well the files have been organized. The brain, however, is more complex than a computer. It is important to note that although some parts of the brain no longer function or may be damaged, other areas of the brain and components of memory will remain in good working order well into the course of many memory loss conditions. However, these working parts must be used regularly to keep them operating to their full capacity for as long as possible.

Types of Memory

The sections that follow discuss a model of memory as a sequence of three stages, from sensory memory, to working/short-term memory, to long-term memory (Figure 1.1).

Working Memory

Working memory, sometimes referred to as short-term memory, is controlled by the central executive system of the brain and comprises three

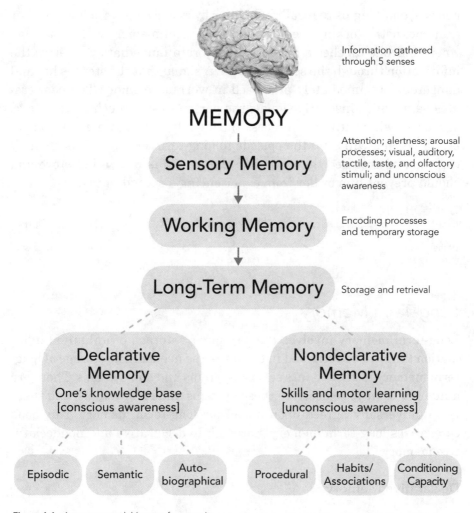

Figure 1.1. A memory model (types of memory).

subsidiary systems: the visuospatial sketchpad, the phonological loop, and the episodic buffer (Baddeley, 2000; Baddeley & Hitch, 1974). The visuospatial sketchpad manipulates and temporarily stores visual and spatial information and images. The phonological loop is the process of rehearsing and understanding auditory information (Baddeley & Hitch, 1974). The episodic buffer combines visual, spatial, and verbal information into episodes and links them to the central executive system in order for the brain to respond appropriately or to move the episodes to long-term memory (Baddeley, 2000). Information in working memory must either be used immediately or moved to long-term memory (Baddeley, 2000). Memories are made as we receive input through our five senses and pay attention to details. We manipulate those details through rehearsal, enabling us to recall them later from our long-term memory. For example, both working memory and long-term memory come into play when someone touches a hot stove. The brain immediately receives the information through the sense of touch. A signal that the stove is hot and dangerous is immediately processed in working memory. The heat creates pain, which instantly signals the person to stop touching the stove. The brain will continue to process the signals, will create an episode to be stored, and will send the episode to long-term memory. This memory can then be accessed the next time the person is near a hot stove and should prevent him or her from experiencing a second injury.

Input	Throughput	Output
Gather details through senses.	Manipulate for storage.	Retrieve the details as needed, and with ease.

Long-Term Memory

Long-term memory involves the permanent storage of unlimited information that can be retrieved in the future as needed. The storage of long-term memory is divided into several systems and sub-systems. There are a number of ways to describe these systems and sub-systems, and there is no universally agreed-upon model for long-term memory. This book categorizes long-term memory storage into declarative and nondeclarative memory.

Declarative Memory

Declarative memory, also referred to as explicit memory, includes episodic, semantic, and autobiographical memory. Episodic memory involves the recollection of events in our lives and the storage of information about the time and place where a particular event occurred. Episodic memory includes remembering facts such as when and where you were born, the name of the first man on the moon, significant historical events, and your location when those events occurred. This type of memory involves relatively conscious, verbal, and intentional recall of specific past experiences or information and words. If you have spent time with a person experiencing memory loss who asked the same question repeatedly, that person is struggling to retrieve details from his or her episodic memory. The person is not intentionally repeating him- or herself, but is seeking information that he or she cannot access (remember) or may not have previously stored in long-term memory.

Another kind of declarative memory is semantic memory, which relates to general factual knowledge that is independent of personal experience. Examples include types of foods, capital cities, and vocabulary. Because people with memory loss have difficulty accessing semantic memory, they become disoriented to time, forget people's names, cannot retain information in conversation, and lose ideas about what to talk about. Individuals with memory loss conditions tend to quickly and easily forget answers to questions that relate to general knowledge.

Finally, autobiographical memory refers to a person's recollection of events and episodes from his or her life and includes both personal semantic and personal episodic memories. Autobiographical memory plays an important role in the formation of identity and self-image and involves a person's subjective and emotional impressions and interpretations of the past (Holland & Kensinger, 2010).

The ability to recall details from declarative memory is increasingly impaired in people with memory loss conditions such as dementia. When a person struggles to remember facts and details from the past, his or her independence is increasingly challenged. A person's ability to recall details about events in history holds less significance than remembering important and basic details related to negotiating his or her way through the day. For example, facts related to finding the bathroom or kitchen need to be accessed from long-term storage several times each day. Facts related to the following are critically important for those with memory loss:

- *Recalling biographical details:* Am I married? Do I have children? Where do I live now?

- *Finding locations:* How do I find the toilet? Where is my bedroom? How do I get home from here?

- *Finding things:* Where are my shoes? Where do I find a coffee mug?

- *Remembering details related to performing tasks:* Did I take my medications today? How many shirts do I need to wear? What type of shirt do I wear today, sleeveless or long-sleeved?

- *Performing tasks in the right order:* I sit before I put on my underwear and socks. I put my underwear on before I put my pants on.

If a person cannot remember these types of facts, care partners need to find a way to help. When required, visual cuing can be incorporated into SR to help those who need extra assistance with recall. Memory aids can also be used to enhance declarative memory and the ability to remember these important details (see the section "Visual Cues and External Memory Aids" in Chapter 3).

Nondeclarative Memory

The second system of long-term memory storage, nondeclarative memory, can also be referred to as implicit memory. This system includes procedural memory, habits and associations, reflexes, and conditioning capacity (the ability to learn through connections between events and stimuli). Nondeclarative memory begins to develop in early childhood and includes habits and skills that are practiced and reinforced through repetition. This type of memory involves unconscious and nonverbal recall of past experiences and is less impaired in people with memory loss conditions such as dementia (Baddeley, 1992). Because this memory system is usually less impaired, nondeclarative memory-based training, such as SR, can be instrumental in helping people to better remember facts and perform actions.

One form of nondeclarative memory is procedural memory, which is the part of long-term memory that is responsible for the habits and associations we use when completing familiar tasks. Procedural memory stores information that helps us complete actions such as washing our hair or driving a car. When driving to a place you travel to often, such as to work or the grocery store, you have probably experienced a time when your mind may have been distracted by other thoughts. While sitting at a stoplight, you may have thought to yourself, "How did I even get here?" Your ability to travel to this point is a result of your procedural memory. You have driven to your specific destination many times, taking the same route in the same way, so that you are now able to do so with very little conscious effort and thought. Another example of procedural memory at work is typing words on a computer keyboard. If you can type without thinking about where the keys are on the keyboard, you have developed the skill through procedural memory. Many activities of daily living are included in this category. When you get dressed each morning, you likely follow a familiar routine, rarely thinking about what you are doing. For example, do you know which foot you put a sock on first? Do you know which leg you put into your pants first? Do you know which side of your mouth you clean first when you brush your teeth? You likely complete these tasks the same way every time. If you have to stop and think about the answers to these questions, these tasks likely take place with little conscious awareness on your part. Habits and associations are built by repeatedly completing a task and reinforcing the steps involved in the process. The more you do something, the better you get at it, and the less you think about the task at hand.

Theoretical Components of Spaced Retrieval

Several theoretical components account for the success of SR, namely classical conditioning, priming, the spacing effect, and errorless learning.

Classical Conditioning

Classical conditioning allows an association to be made between a lead question and a response, a key step in the SR process (see Chapter 2), by taking advantage of implicit memory, which is preserved in many people who have memory loss (Camp, Foss, O'Hanlon, & Stevens, 1996; Camp & Stevens, 1990). Natural reinforcement is provided as the rate of successful practice increases (Bjork, 1988). Pavlov (1897/1902) first introduced classical conditioning when he noticed that dogs, who were being studied for other purposes, began to salivate when the scientists entered the room with food. He noticed that they salivated before they were given the food. This phenomenon became known as classical conditioning and proved that a reaction can be created based on a previous action (Huitt & Hummel, 1997). Scientists have since shown that this reaction is part of unconscious memory. For example, if someone with memory loss encountered a person who was upsetting or argumentative in the past, a subsequent invitation to spend time with that person may elicit a negative response or be distressing even if he or she does not consciously recall the conflict. A care partner can change this association by beginning with a positive experience (e.g., invite the person to sit with you over a cup of coffee or tea) and thereby decondition the negative response. SR's effectiveness is founded on this scientific principle. The SR strategy integrates positive reinforcement by asking the same lead question while increasing the amount of time before asking again. Each time the person successfully practices the response, he or she is naturally rewarded for the successful response, and new behaviors are shaped (Bjork, 1988).

Priming

Priming is an unconscious form of memory that involves activating particular representations or associations in memory just before carrying out a task. In other words, one action prompts the next action. Many basic life-sustaining activities and self-care skills can be learned through priming. For example, we learn to accept food from a fork when it is placed next to our mouth. The action of loading a fork with food and moving it toward the mouth prompts us to open our mouth and take a bite. Similarly, picking up a hairbrush prompts you to brush your hair.

Priming can occur automatically, or it can be established through practice (Posner & Snyder, 1975). People with memory loss can benefit from the effects of priming even if they cannot remember using or practicing the information (Squire, 1992). SR takes advantage of priming in several ways. First, a lead question and response are established for use during practice. The lead question and response are related, and the response has been relevant to the person at some point in the past, which will help the person to recognize the response more quickly (Collins & Loftus, 1975). Second, SR takes advantage of the unconscious nature of the learning because the lead question prompts the expected response. The care partner asks the lead question and expects the person with memory loss to produce the response right away, or the care partner provides the response. The person with memory loss is, therefore, not required to actively remember the association between the lead question and response and instead relies on unconscious memory and prompting during SR practice.

The Spacing Effect

The spacing effect is based on the finding that information is learned and retrieved more effectively when practices are spaced over time compared to learning that is practiced repeatedly within a short amount of time (Baddeley, 1999; Wilson, 2009), or a consecutive or massed practice of learning information (Balota, Duchek, & Logan, 2007; Neath & Surprenant, 2003). Memory and successful recall increase when the timing between the practice of information is spaced in a systematic way, even for those with cognitive impairment. SR was designed around the spacing effect by having the care partner create successive practices at increasing time intervals.

In his study of human memory, Ebbinghaus (1913) established the underpinnings for the modern use of SR by applying the spacing effect to learning new information. Using himself as his only subject, Ebbinghaus presented a series of six to eight previously unknown nonsense syllables for memorization, waited a predetermined amount of time, and then retested himself to measure how much he was able to retain. He set the mastery criterion for learning during memorization at two consecutive error-free recalls to ensure that a correct recall was not accidental. Once he was successful, he implemented retention intervals by increasing the intervals from several minutes up to 31 days to ensure he would continue to recall the information. He defined retention intervals for his research as the point following the last memorization until testing. After the retention interval, Ebbinghaus (1913) tested his memory by relearning the stimuli (previously unknown nonsense syllables) used at memorization. He found that he required fewer trials to relearn the syllables with each subsequent retention interval, which he defined as savings. Since this study, many researchers have examined the best type of interval for effective learning and recall (Glenberg, 1977; Peterson, Wampler, Kirkpatrick, & Saltzman, 1963; Spitzer, 1939). Research has repeatedly confirmed that presenting learning opportunities over expanding time intervals, instead of massed practice, improves learning. SR's effectiveness is founded on this scientific principle because time intervals are expanded when the learner provides a correct response and are reduced when the learner provides an incorrect response.

Memory Outcomes with Errorless Learning

Errorless learning contributes to the likelihood of increased long-term retention and supports learning the correct response by eliminating errors as well as the process of searching to find the response during practice (Fridriksson, Holland, Beeson, & Morrow, 2005; Turkstra & Bourgeois, 2005). SR is considered an errorless learning strategy because the lead question and response are timed and structured so as to prevent incorrect answers as much as possible. Research has shown that people with memory impairment learn more effectively in situations where errors are prevented (Wilson, Baddeley, Evans, & Shiel, 1994). Therefore, practice of new information should include as few errors as possible (Baddeley, 1992; Wilson et al., 1994), because people with explicit memory deficits cannot recall personal episodes (episodic memory) and consequently cannot use the past as a basis for improving or self-correcting. However, if errors are minimized, the opportunity to learn information accurately is increased.

Errorless learning can be integrated into procedures that focus on enhancing abilities and self-esteem. People with memory loss too often experience the constant impact of failure. The combination of constant failure with increasing loss of ability negatively impacts self-esteem. The errorless learning approach eliminates opportunities for learning the incorrect information while teaching the correct information in a way that sets the person up for successful outcomes. Errorless learning is incorporated into the framework of SR by instituting short and increasing intervals of time between practices of information while also reducing the time between intervals if the person was not successful. This kind of interval spacing immediately provides an opportunity for the person to experience success. In addition to manipulating time intervals, the care partner implementing SR can also provide the correct answer to the lead question when

- The person is struggling to find the answer
- The person answers incorrectly
- The person is unable to answer at all

Incrementally increasing time intervals and eliminating opportunities to learn incorrect information contribute to errorless learning (Baddeley, 1992; Jokel, Rochon, & Anderson, 2010; Wilson et al., 1994). These strategies support the aim of SR by teaching the person the information he or she needs for long-term use while also focusing on successful outcomes.

— — — — — — — —

This overview of memory provides the foundation upon which SR is built. The next chapter outlines a practical, step-by-step process for implementing SR with people experiencing memory loss. Having an understanding of why and how SR works enables care partners to determine how to implement the intervention most effectively to meet an individual's needs.

CHAPTER 2
Putting Spaced Retrieval into Practice

This chapter walks you through each step of the Spaced Retrieval (SR) process. Each step is equally important and should be completed in the sequence presented in order for the SR intervention to be successful. These recommendations have been compiled following careful consideration of how SR has been used in clinical practice and research (see Chapter 5 for a summary of published research on SR).

The SR steps are as follows:

Step 1. Identify the person's need or desire.

Step 2. Conduct an SR screening using the Spaced Retrieval Screening Form to determine if the person is responsive to SR. Complete the Reading Screening Form if you are incorporating a continuous visual cue into the SR practice or using SR to teach the use of an external memory aid.

Step 3. Develop a lead question and response and implement the practice intervals.

Step 4. Modify the SR procedure when needed and reinforce the information the person learned.

The sections that follow discuss each step in detail to lay the foundation for success in using SR.

Identify the Person's Need or Desire

The first step when preparing to implement SR is to identify the person's need or desire. A need is something that is very important; it is necessary or required. A desire is a wish or a want. Both are key elements of well-being and should be considered when making decisions about the focus of your goals for supporting memory and behavior. For example, a person may need to remember not to bear weight on a broken foot or may desire to remember the date of her wedding anniversary. Someone with memory loss still has the same desires as others. The person desires to socialize, express needs, participate in hobbies, interact with family, be included in activities, teach and learn, and enjoy being asked for advice. The person has the same desire to contribute to the household or the community. The need to communicate and to be productive does not end once a person begins to experience the challenges associated with memory loss. As the person struggles to communicate and remember daily information, he or she needs to have conversations and relationships that are meaningful and successful.

Take a moment to imagine not being able to remember why you are not living in your own home with your spouse. Every morning, a stranger comes into your room to help you bathe and get dressed. Now, imagine that you cannot think of the word "husband" and you are having trouble expressing the feeling of missing your spouse. How would you feel? What might you do? Most likely you would feel frustrated, or perhaps embarrassed or inadequate. Worse, you might start refusing help. You might use gestures and words that may not make sense to others in an effort to communicate.

Sometimes those who struggle with memory loss conditions have a reputation for displaying challenging or disruptive behaviors. While these behaviors might be perceived as negative, they tend to be a means of communicating unmet needs. In fact, these behaviors are often referred to as *responsive behaviors*, a term that places the focus on the unmet need rather than on the person who is causing the perceived problem. The unmet need is the trigger, not the person. Furthermore, when addressed properly, the behaviors are a mechanism for interactive communication between care partners and the person with memory loss. When we imagine ourselves in someone else's place and try to view the world through his or her eyes, we are better able to interpret responsive behaviors.

Knowing the person with memory loss will help you to figure out what the person needs and desires. Make an effort to speak with the person's family and find out where he or she lived, what he or she did for a living, and what he or she enjoyed doing, including hobbies and interests. Ask about favorite foods, songs, movies, and so forth. The more you can learn about the person, the more you will have to talk about and the easier it will be to assist the person when he or she has difficulty communicating a need or desire. When you witness a behavior that you may not understand, begin by asking yourself, Why is this behavior happening? When is this happening? When is this not happening? Is the person afraid? Hungry? Bored? Experiencing pain? Would the person like to go outside, sit with her husband, or be able to remember where she lives?

Care partners through the implementation of SR can be instrumental in helping to fulfill a person's needs and desires. SR allows the person with memory loss to experience positive reinforcement and successful outcomes that clearly illustrate that he or she is still able to complete tasks and remember important details and information. When implementing SR, it is important for care partners to realize that there are still many tasks the person with memory loss can do if supports are put in place. Care partners will have the most success when they encourage and support skills that remain rather than focus on impaired abilities. Researchers and clinicians have used SR to address many different responsive behaviors, desires to complete tasks, or needs to remember information to increase safety. The following selection of memory goals for Safety, Activities of Daily Living and Independence, Orientation and Wayfinding, and Details and Information are taken from research and clinical use of the SR practice.

⊕ Safety

- Following through with emergency procedures (e.g., what to do when injured, shouting for help in public)
- Using the call button for assistance in the bedroom
- Using an emergency alert system when home alone
- Calling 911 in an emergency
- Locking wheelchair brakes before standing
- Transferring safely from a chair or bed
- Using a walker or assistive device
- Holding the handrail when using stairs
- Using a compensatory swallow strategy to improve safety during meals

Activities of Daily Living and Independence

- Remembering to use a calendar to complete daily activities
- Recalling daily tasks

- Using a schedule or other external memory aid
- Following the steps for dressing, toileting, or brushing teeth
- Washing hands after using the toilet
- Turning on/off lights upon entering/exiting a room
- Using a cell phone
- Eating independently
- Following step-by-step directions for household tasks, such as doing laundry
- Putting dirty clothes in a hamper
- Taking medication on time
- Asking for pain medication when uncomfortable
- Completing daily chores

🕐 Orientation and Wayfinding

- Recalling room number, phone number, or address
- Recalling how to find the bathroom or dining room
- Learning where to look to find certain information, such as the answer to a frequently asked question (e.g., when he or she is going home, when a spouse is coming to visit, or when a meal will be served)

📝 Details and Information

- Recognizing someone's face and recalling his or her name
- Addressing someone by name
- Naming people from pictures
- Naming household objects
- Naming pills
- Recalling target information over the telephone (e.g., medication times and room numbers)
- Repeating instructions

- Remembering meaningful recent events

- Completing cued recall of behavior

- Reaching goals (e.g., increase conversation skills and activity participation, decrease repetitive questions)

- Referring to or conversing with the use of a memory book

Once needs and desires are identified, the care partner will choose one concept or physical task for the SR process. Typically, the person's safety is addressed first to avoid unwanted injury and further complications. Consider what the person really needs to remember as an outcome of SR training and then keep goals functional, concrete, and relevant to the person.

Spaced Retrieval Screening

Before implementing SR, it is recommended that you complete a Spaced Retrieval screening to determine whether the person is an appropriate candidate for SR (Brush & Camp, 1998c). The Spaced Retrieval Screening Form is used to identify those individuals who are able to retain a piece of novel information for 30 seconds. An individual may not be an appropriate candidate for SR if he or she is unable to recall information after a 30-second interval after three attempts. To date, several researchers have successfully implemented the SR screening procedure into their SR studies (Benigas & Bourgeois, in press; Bourgeois et al., 2003; Hickey & How, 2008; Joltin, Camp, & McMahon, 2003; Small, 2012).

Use the Spaced Retrieval Screening Form to record the details of each practice. Record the time interval that was used, and mark if the response was correct, incorrect, or not provided at all. There is also a space to keep any relevant notes during each practice. For example, maybe the dog began to bark right after the lead question was presented, and the individual provided the wrong response. This level of distraction should be noted and provides a reasonable explanation as to why an incorrect response may have been given. Most of the time, however, there will be nothing to record as to why either an incorrect response or no response at all was given, and that is perfectly fine. The care partner who will be using SR should conduct the screening in a quiet location with minimal distractions. Turn off the TV or radio and close the blinds, if necessary. If family members or other care partners are present, ask them to remain quiet during the screening and to refrain from offering any assistance. To see completed Spaced Retrieval Screening Forms used in a variety of case examples, refer to Chapter 4. The steps of the SR screening process are as follows.

Five Easy Spaced Retrieval Screening Steps

1. Choose novel information to the individual (e.g., your name, if the person doesn't know you).

2. Choose the response that you will use in the screening (e.g., Lisa).

3. Choose a lead question that you will ask (e.g., What is my name?).

4. Make sure the person understands the question and the expected answer.

5. Implement practice beginning with a 5-second delay, advancing to 10 seconds, then 20 seconds, and ending with 30 seconds.

If at any time the individual makes three consecutive errors, the care partner should stop the screening and attempt again on another day. If the person provides the correct response during the immediate practice, advance to a 5-second delay. If the response is correct, advance to a 10-second delay, then 20 seconds, and ending with a 30-second delay. If an incorrect response is provided, return to the last successful time delay.

Conducting the Spaced Retrieval Screening

The following case study example demonstrates the SR screening procedure in practice.

 Meet Ron

Ron lives in a long-term care community. He has always stayed in a private room, but recently the staff moved him to a new room where he now has a roommate. The staff has noticed that he is unable to remember his new roommate. As a result, he occasionally becomes aggressive and states, "This guy won't go home." The staff wants to find a way to decrease his responsive behaviors for increased safety and decreased stress for both residents when Ron gets upset. Staff feel that SR may be the best strategy to teach Ron that he has a roommate, but they would like to complete a screening to determine if success is likely before implementing an SR practice (see the sample SR Screening Form for Ron).

Spaced Retrieval Screening Form

Name: *Ron* Date: *May 5th*

Lead Question: *What is my name?*

Response: *Lisa*

Goal: *30 Seconds*

Practice Trial	Time Interval	Correct Response?			Notes
		Yes	No	NR	
1	5s	X			
2	10s	X			
3	20s	X			
4	30s		X		
5	20s	X			
6	30s	X			

*NR=no response

As Lisa, Ron's nursing assistant, worked with Ron, she tracked his progress on a Spaced Retrieval Screening Form (see the sample portion of the form). Ron provided the correct response during the first three practices, but then demonstrated some difficulty during the fourth practice. Lisa provided the correct answer, asked Ron for an immediate response, and then reduced the time interval to that of the last successful practice. By the sixth practice, Ron was able to remember Lisa's name after a 30-second interval, an indication that he could be a viable candidate for SR (see the dialogue exchange between Lisa and Ron).

At times, a care partner may find that the SR screening does not go as smoothly as the case example provided. After three consecutive errors have been made, the SR screening should be discontinued and attempted again on a different day. People with memory loss conditions have good days and bad days, so one failure does not mean that SR will never be a good strategy to use with that individual. If someone has failed three consecutive times during the SR screening, it is important to conclude in an upbeat and positive manner. You might say something like, "I can tell you are trying very hard to remember my name, and I really appreciate the effort you are making. Since we both have a lot of important things to get done today, I think that is enough practice for now. We will work on it again tomorrow."

Lisa:	I would like to help you remember my name. My name is Lisa *(Lisa points to her name tag.) (No time delay; immediate memory response expected)* Ron, what is my name?
Ron:	Lisa.
Lisa:	That's right. We're going to keep trying to remember that. *(5-second delay)* Ron, what is my name?
Ron:	Lisa.
Lisa:	That's right. Let's see if you can remember it for a little longer this time. *(10-second delay)* Ron, what is my name?
Ron:	Lisa.
Lisa:	Good. Let's keep practicing. *(20-second delay)* Ron, what is my name?
Ron:	Lisa.
Lisa:	That's right. I want you to remember even longer now. *(30-second delay)* Ron, what is my name?
Ron:	It's not the same name as my daughter's.
Lisa:	You know what Ron? You're right. Your daughter and I have different names. My name is Lisa. What is my name?
Ron:	Lisa.
Lisa:	That's right. Let's try it again because I think you're getting it. *(20-second delay)* Ron, what is my name?
Ron:	Lisa.
Lisa:	Great job, Ron! You will be remembering my name in no time at all. *(30-second delay)* Ron, what is my name?
Ron:	Lisa.
Lisa:	You did a fantastic job remembering my name. Now let's work on something else.

If an individual is unable to get through the screening with success, he or she is unlikely to experience success with SR, and nothing else needs to be completed. If the person does successfully complete the screening, you can then move on to conduct the reading screening.

Reading Screening

Note that because visual aids are often incorporated into SR training, it is important to conduct a separate screening to determine if the individual can read, what type size is the most appropriate, and if the person comprehends what has been read (more information about visual aids can be found in Chapter 3). The care partner can initiate a reading screening at the same time as the SR screening or when a complete evaluation of the person's abilities is conducted. Since SR can be implemented with or without a visual aid, individuals who are unable to read or see can also benefit from this intervention. Use the Reading Screening Form to record relevant information related to reading and the details of each reading trial. On the second page of the Reading Screening Form is a sentence reading tool that the care partner can use to determine at what type size the person with memory loss is most comfortable reading. For an example of a completed Reading Screening Form, see the case example of Mr. Farmer in Chapter 4. The directions that follow can be used to implement the reading screening.

Six Easy Reading Screening Steps

1. Ask the individual to help you determine the best size of type that he or she can comfortably read.

2. Have the individual hold the page with the sentences in his or her nondominant hand.

3. Starting at the top of the page, point to one sentence at a time. Say, "Read the sentence aloud and then do what it says." Record the person's responses on the Reading Screening Form.

4. Place the person's name and room number sign on a wall 48–60 inches off the ground (use the lower height if the person is in a wheelchair).

5. Position the individual 10 feet away from the sign.

6. Ask the individual to read the sign aloud, and then record the person's response.

Develop a Lead Question and Response

After completing the relevant screenings, the next step is for the care partner to develop the lead question and response based on the identified need or desire. Lead questions should be simple and direct, and the person with memory loss should understand what is being asked. The answer, or the response, should be short, to the point, and result in the concept or physical task that needs to be recalled and/or performed. The less the person with memory loss is asked to recall, the more success he or she will experience. Neither the lead question nor response should be confusing for the care partner to ask or the person with memory loss to answer. They should be simple enough to easily incorporate into everyday dialogue and should include vocabulary and terminology that the person would have chosen and used (see case example of Mr. Farmer in Chapter 4 for an example of how to choose appropriate terminology in SR practice). Only one lead question and response should be used at a time during practice. See the examples of lead questions and responses in Figure 2.1.

Implement the Spaced Retrieval Procedures

A care partner can begin using SR after the screenings are completed and the lead question and response are chosen. When getting started with the intervention, care partners should never assume that the individual understands why he or she is engaging in the activity. Take a few moments to ensure that the person understands what will be expected of him or her. Based on our examination of the practical implementation of SR in research and clinical practice, we recommend the following steps for getting started.

Four Easy Education Steps

1. Tell the person what is going to be learned and why.

2. Introduce the lead question and response. If a physical task is required, demonstrate it and make sure the person can perform it.

3. If using a continuous visual cue during practice, introduce it at this time. Make sure the person can read it and understands what it says. Place it in the person's direct line of sight, show him or her where it will be located, and say, "You can look at this whenever you have trouble remembering the information during practice." (Chapter 3 discusses continuous visual cues in detail.)

4. Immediately ask the lead question and allow the person to answer with the response. If a physical task is being taught, ask him or her to perform it.

Safety

What should you do every time you take a drink? *Sip, tuck, and swallow*

What should you do after you take a bite of food? *Take a drink*

What should you do when you are finished eating? *Clean my mouth out with my finger OR Wipe my mouth*

What should you do before you stand up from your wheelchair? *Lock the brakes*

How do you stand up safely? *Put my hands on the chair or bed and push up*

How do you sit down safely? *Reach back for the chair or bed and sit down slowly*

What do you need to use every time you walk? *My cane*

How do you walk safely when using your walker? *Keep my feet inside the walker OR Keep the walker on the floor*

How do you get help when you are in your room? *I press the red button*

What should you do if you fall in your house and need help? *Push the button on my necklace*

Activities of Daily Living and Independence

What should you do when you want to find the toilet? *Follow the arrow*

When you take off your clothes, where should you put them? *In the laundry basket*

Where do you keep your clothes? *In the closet*

Where do you keep your underwear? *In my dresser*

Where do you keep your glasses? *On my bedside table*

What should you do before you go to breakfast in the morning? *Rinse my dentures and put them in my mouth*

What should you do before you go to bed? *Take out my dentures and put them in the cup*

Orientation and Wayfinding

Where should you look when you want to know what day it is? *My calendar*

What is your address? *123 Main Street*

What building do you live in? *Fireside Manor*

What is your room number? *416*

What should you look for when you want to find your room? *My picture next to the door*

What floor do you live on? *4th floor*

What number do you press in the elevator to go home? *4*

Details and Information

What is your daughter's name? *Katie*

What is the name of the woman who comes to help you shower? *Mary*

Where should you look when you want to know when your husband is coming to visit? *My calendar*

Where should you look when you want to know what you are doing today? *My schedule*

Figure 2.1. Sample lead questions and responses.

How to Get Started

The following case example of Victor demonstrates how to begin implementing SR.

 Meet Victor

Jerry is a home care coordinator who speaks with his clients on the phone regularly, but only sees them face to face once or twice a month, so it is hard for him to implement SR. His client Victor lives at home with his wife Rosemary. Victor has vascular dementia and often forgets that a care partner comes to their home each day for a few hours. As a result, when the care partner knocks on the door and asks to be let in the house, Victor tells her to go home and will not let her enter.

Four Easy Steps for Jerry and Victor

1. Victor's desire: To feel safe about who he is letting in the house.

2. Victor's need: To have help with daily chores, such as meal preparation and cleaning.

3. The lead question Jerry will ask Victor (when shown a picture of the care partner): "What do you do when Ellen knocks on the door?"

4. Victor's response will be: "Let her in."

Jerry arranged to visit one day when Ellen, the care partner, would be in Victor's home. Jerry gave Ellen a large-print nametag to wear on her coat. He took a picture of Ellen wearing her coat and nametag standing in front of Victor's house and added a caption: "Ellen comes to cook our meals. When she knocks, I open the door and let her in." Jerry explained to Victor that Ellen stops by frequently to help with meals and that together they would practice learning who she is so that Victor would remember to let her into the home. Jerry showed Victor the picture of Ellen and made sure he was able to read the caption below the photo. Jerry placed the external memory aid on the inside of the door and showed Victor where it would be located. Next, he introduced the lead question and response by saying, "This is Ellen. When she knocks on the door, let her in." Jerry then immediately asked the lead question, "What do you do when Ellen knocks on the door?" and allowed Victor to immediately respond, "Let her in." Jerry asked Victor to practice looking at Ellen's picture and opening the door.

After the person has been introduced to the lead question and appropriate response and understands the purpose of performing the activity, practice sessions can begin. Practice sessions should last 30–60 minutes. Researchers and clinicians have successfully used a variety of time intervals to help the person learn the response. In this chapter, we provide a practice schedule that details how to structure the time intervals as the person with memory loss successfully responds.

First Spaced Retrieval Practice Session

When conducting the first SR practice session, refer to the four basic steps that follow.

Four Easy Implementation Steps

1. Follow the four easy education steps outlined earlier: explain what the person will be learning and why, introduce the lead question and response, demonstrate any physical task expected of the person, and introduce any visual cue (if used).

2. If the person provides the response during the immediate practice, advance the time interval according to the practice schedule. The time interval should begin after the person performs the physical task.

3. If the person provides an incorrect answer, provide the correct response, redirect him or her to the continuous visual cue (if using one), and try again.

4. If the person answers incorrectly during three consecutive practices, stop the session and try again on a different day.

All Subsequent Spaced Retrieval Practice Sessions

You can structure each subsequent SR practice session using the following steps.

Four Easy Implementation Steps

1. Begin each session by measuring learning progress. Without any practice, ask the lead question and allow the person to answer with the response immediately. If a physical task is required (e.g., locking wheelchair brakes, crossing off items on a schedule, using a compensatory swallow strategy), ask the person to perform it while or after he or she provides the response. It is important to confirm that the person is learning the physical task and not simply learning the response of reading the continuous visual cue. For this reason, we recommend not introducing the continuous visual cue for practice until after this step is completed.

2. If the person provides the response and performs any physical tasks required, make note of the success by saying "That's right," "Very good," or "Well done" and advance the time interval according to the practice schedule. The time interval should begin after the response is given and the physical task is performed.

3. If the person answers incorrectly, repeat the lead question and response procedures. Keep errorless learning in mind and do not tell the person that he or she was wrong or made a mistake. Simply provide the correct response, keeping your tone informative and the correction brief. Once the person is able to provide the response and immediately perform any physical task, advance the time interval according to the practice schedule. The time interval should begin after the response is given and the physical task is performed.

4. When the person is able to provide the response at the beginning of three consecutive sessions without any formalized practice between sessions, the information is considered learned and stored in long-term memory. However, some additional practices may be required to help with generalization, or the performance of the task independently and outside of practices.

The following practice schedule can be used to structure each SR practice session over the course of the training.

Practice Schedule

1. First, elicit an immediate response along with the performance of the physical task (if the person's response includes one).

2. Use the following intervals when advancing or decreasing time:
    5 seconds (s)→10s→20s→30s→1 minute (min)→2 min→4 min→8 min→16 min

3. Each time the correct response is provided and physical task performed, advance to the next time interval by waiting to ask the lead question. The time interval should begin after the response is given and the physical task is performed.

4. Each time an incorrect response is provided, redirect the person to the continuous visual cue (if using one), provide the correct response, ask the lead question, and have the person answer immediately and perform the physical task. Then, decrease the time interval by half before asking the lead question again. The time interval should begin after the response is given and the physical task is performed.

5. During time intervals, the person can engage in a pleasurable activity or conversation or work toward another goal unrelated to what is being taught through SR. Clinicians and family members have filled the time between practice intervals with games, reading, exercise, walking, eating, music, and activities of daily living. The choice of activity is not important as long as it is pleasing or interesting to the person and unrelated to SR. If the activities are related to what is being taught, it may take longer to reach the desired outcome because the response is being continually activated and not stored for later retrieval. It is recommended that you wait to introduce activities until the 2-minute time interval has been successfully reached. As previously noted, most practice sessions last 30–60 minutes.

6. Use the Spaced Retrieval Data Form provided in this chapter to track the relevant information from each practice session.

Learning Where to Find Important Items

The case example that follows demonstrates SR practice sessions in action as well as how SR might be implemented in the home setting.

 Meet Gina

Gina lives at home with her husband Bill. She has always kept her glasses in a basket on the kitchen table, but after having a recent stroke, she never seems to be able to remember where they are. She often worries that she has lost her glasses, so she asks Bill several times throughout the day, "Do you know where my glasses are?" Bill will use SR to help Gina practice remembering where to find her glasses. Soon, she will not have to ask Bill about her glasses anymore and will remember where they are located.

Five Easy Steps for Gina and Bill

1. Gina's need: to remember the location of her glasses.

2. The lead question Bill will ask Gina: "Where do you keep your glasses?"

3. Gina's response will be: "On the kitchen table."

4. Bill will walk over to the kitchen table with Gina to make sure she sees and understands that her glasses are there.

5. Bill will help Gina to practice remembering where to find her glasses (as shown in their dialogue exchange).

> **Bill:** I would like to help you remember that you keep your glasses right here on the kitchen table. *(Bill shows Gina the glasses.)* Gina, where do you keep your glasses?
>
> **Gina:** On the kitchen table.
>
> **Bill:** That's right. We are going to keep trying to remember that. Gina, where do you keep your glasses?
>
> **Gina:** I think they are over here by the couch.
>
> **Bill:** Your glasses are on the kitchen table. *(Bill shows Gina the glasses.)* Gina, where do you keep your glasses?

Bill will continue to ask Gina where she keeps her glasses using the recommended SR schedule (5s, 10s, 20s, 30s, 1 min, 2 min, 4 min, 8 min, and 16 min). After 2 minutes, Bill turns on Gina's favorite television show while the time intervals pass. Once Bill reaches 16 minutes between asking the lead question, he will take a break and try again later in the day or the next day until Gina is remembering where she keeps her glasses all by herself.

— — — — — — — —

Each person with memory loss will respond to SR in different ways. We recommend using the Spaced Retrieval Data Form during each practice session. The form will allow the care partner to track progress and to make decisions whether to modify or terminate practice based on how the individual has performed. Success will look different for each individual. The overall goal is to help the person recall the information being taught for improved independence, safety, and quality of life; however, successfully achieving the goal will vary. Careful data collection of the practice outcomes can help gauge success. For example, in some cases a person will make frequent errors and rely on use of the continuous visual cue for every practice. As the person participates in more practice sessions, he or she may advance more quickly through the time intervals or rely on the continuous visual cue less. This indicates progress and can motivate the care team to keep going (see Chapter 3 for information about including the care team in SR practice). In a situation where a care partner is billing for treatment, the Spaced Retrieval Data Form will support progress. During each practice, the time interval should be recorded, and reliance on the continuous visual cue should be noted. The care partner should mark if the verbal response was correct, incorrect, or not given at all in addition to marking if the physical task was performed correctly. At times, the individual may give the correct verbal response, but not perform the physical task. Remember that both are important in achieving the end goal. Figure 2.2 outlines each step of the Spaced Retrieval practice.

How and When to Modify the SR Procedure

At times, the care partner may find that a person with memory loss successfully completed the SR screening but is not succeeding during practice. This can be frustrating. Fortunately, SR can be adapted to meet the needs of the person. Because cognition and responsiveness in someone with a memory loss condition can differ day to day, try the step-by-step procedure for several practice sessions before implementing any modifications. While there are no standard protocols for how and when to change elements of the SR model, we as well as many other researchers and clinicians have found that adjustments to several different variables can still lead to successful practices. We recommend only changing one variable at a time and implementing the changed variable across several practice sessions before deeming it either successful or ineffective. For a detailed example of how to adapt SR when progress is slow, see the case example of Jack in Chapter 4.

Modification Suggestions to Address Failure

When a person with memory loss struggles to learn information using SR, modifying the lead question, response, or time interval can be effective in helping the individual to address failure during practice sessions.

Modify the Lead Question

Adjust the way the lead question is asked or shorten its length. If changes are made, teach the person the new lead question and then make sure that you ask the new lead question during practice sessions. Be careful not to accidentally return to using the old lead question or vocabulary. Consider the following when evaluating the lead question:

- Is the lead question too confusing for the person to answer?
- Does the lead question prompt the response in a natural way?
- Is the lead question relevant to the person?
- Is the need or desire that the lead question addresses functional?
- Is the lead question concrete and simple?
- Does the lead question use familiar words?

Modify the Response

Adjust what the person is expected to say and do or shorten the length of the response. Whenever the response is modified, make sure the continuous visual cue also reflects the change, and educate the person using the new response. Consider the following when evaluating the response:

- Is the response vocabulary part of the person's normal repertoire (e.g., notebook or journal)?
- Is the response relevant to the person?
- Do the response and related physical task require little cognitive or physical effort?
- Is the response concrete and simple?

SPACED RETRIEVAL STEP BY STEP

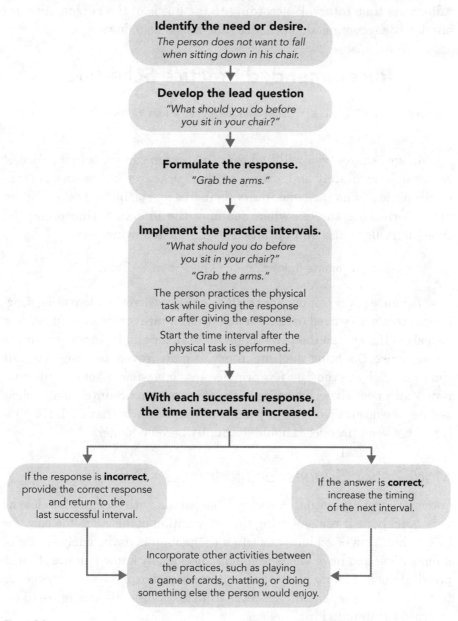

Identify the need or desire.
The person does not want to fall when sitting down in his chair.

Develop the lead question
"What should you do before you sit in your chair?"

Formulate the response.
"Grab the arms."

Implement the practice intervals.
"What should you do before you sit in your chair?"

"Grab the arms."

The person practices the physical task while giving the response or after giving the response.

Start the time interval after the physical task is performed.

With each successful response, the time intervals are increased.

If the response is **incorrect**, provide the correct response and return to the last successful interval.

If the answer is **correct**, increase the timing of the next interval.

Incorporate other activities between the practices, such as playing a game of cards, chatting, or doing something else the person would enjoy.

Figure 2.2.

Modify the Time Intervals

Adjust the time intervals according to the needs of the person. As a reminder, the recommended practice schedule is as follows:

Recommended Practice Schedule

5 seconds (s)→10s→20s→30s→1 minute (min)→2 min→4 min→8 min→16 min

---

In some cases, you will find that the person can provide the correct response immediately and after very short practices but begins to experience difficulty as the time intervals increase. For individuals who are not experiencing success when doubling the intervals, shortening the time intervals is also appropriate, such as the following:

1 minute (min)→2 min→3 min→5 min→8 min

Because a key component of SR's success is errorless learning, practice intervals may need to be adjusted to eliminate incorrect responses or periods of time when the person is searching for and trying to formulate the response. Doubling the time intervals may provide too long of a wait time, especially in the first few practice sessions when all of the information is still new. Experimenting with different practice intervals to elicit success is encouraged. The key point to remember is that each time interval between practices should gradually become longer.

Modification Suggestions to Increase Difficulty

You may encounter situations where the person with memory loss learns very quickly, as if remembering the information using SR is too easy for him or her. This often happens when the person is in the early stages of memory loss and he or she is practicing previously known information or physical tasks. Modifying the time intervals and expanding the response to be more complex can increase the difficulty of the SR procedure to accommodate an individual's needs.

Modify the Time Intervals

If the person is very successful at recalling previously learned information or learning a new physical task, using the typical shorter time intervals may seem annoying, senseless, or distracting to the person. For individuals who learn quickly, expanding the time intervals to greater lengths may be appropriate, such as the following:

1 minute (min)→2 min→6 min→10 min→16 min

Again, no matter what interval is chosen, the critical factor is to make each time interval longer than the previous one used if the interval has been successful.

Increase Expectations

If SR has been a very effective tool for teaching new information, the care partner may wish to build on the success achieved during practice. This can be accomplished by expanding the existing response to become more complex. Although useful, this type of modification may not be appropriate for everyone, as the responses can become long and difficult to recall without cognitive effort. Consider using a longer response when teaching multi-step tasks, such as self-care activities or compensatory strategies to improve safety during eating. It is important to practice one response at a time. Be sure the person has learned the response (correct recall at first practice, without additional reinforcement and education, over three consecutive sessions) before making it more difficult. When the first part of the response has been learned, begin practicing on the second part. Make sure to add the new part of the response to the continuous visual cue and educate the person on the added steps accordingly (see Figure 2.3). Continue this pattern until all parts of the response are learned.

Below are three steps that can be used to teach a person with memory loss how to dress the lower half of his or her body. In this example, the lead question stays the same throughout all parts of SR training:

Lead question for each response part: What should you do after you put on your shirt in the morning?

Response part 1: Put on my underwear.

Response part 2: Put on my underwear and then my pants.

Response part 3: Put on my underwear, then my pants, and then my belt last.

For more complex, multi-step tasks, it might not be realistic to have the person perform each physical task during each practice. In the dressing example, it would be very time-consuming and physically taxing to ask the person to repeatedly dress and undress. However, since motor learn-

Put on my underwear.

Put on my underwear
and then my pants.

Put on my underwear,
then my pants,
and my belt last.

Figure 2.3. Modify the continuous visual cue to reflect the response.

ing involves preserved implicit memory, it is recommended that the person perform part of a physical task during practices and that he or she execute the full task at the end of the practice session. For instance, a person who is remembering how to get dressed can put on his or her belt each time and then perform the entire procedure after the last practice. A belt was chosen in this example because in independent performance outside of practice sessions, if the first two steps are missed, the person will have nowhere to put the belt. This signals to the person that some steps have been forgotten and might help him or her to remember to put on the underwear and pants. For a more detailed example of how to teach a multi-step process using SR, see the case example of Mrs. Tech in Chapter 4.

When to Stop Spaced Retrieval

There are no formal recommendations for when to stop making modifications and discontinue SR because every person will learn at a different rate. Existing research shows that some people can find success with SR after one practice session (Bird, Alexopoulos, & Adamowicz, 1995), whereas for others, it might take up to more than 30 practice sessions (Benigas & Bourgeois, in press). Be sure not to give up too soon, as the person may need a lot of time to learn what is being taught. The care partner needs to consider several factors before deciding when to discontinue the practice:

- Have tasks been modified to increase the likelihood of success? For example, was a continuous visual cue incorporated into the practice sessions? If the person was challenged by longer time intervals, were they broken into increases that are more gradual?

- Is the person making any progress at all? Everyone achieves improvement at different rates. Refer back to the Spaced Retrieval Data Form to see if progress has been made. Even small gains can be counted as progress.

- Is the person showing signs of frustration or anger? If the person asks the care partner to "stop bothering" him or her, it is probably time to end the practices.

- Are other members of the care team reinforcing the practices? Once the other members of the care team are consistently reinforcing the SR practice, the care partner who implemented SR can usually stop the practice if it is part of a treatment plan (see Chapter 3 for more information).

- Is the continuous visual cue accessible and meaningful? The person needs to be able to see the continuous visual cue and know that it can be relied on for success.

- Has the person met the mastery criterion by incorporating the new information or physical task into his or her daily routine? Once the person is automatically performing the task or habitually recalling the information in daily life, he or she has reached the SR goal.

Reinforce the Spaced Retrieval Practice to Facilitate Learning

After the person has achieved his or her goal through the SR training, it is essential to continue monitoring the recall of information and performance of any physical tasks. Reinforce the information learned in SR as you continue to support the person's needs and desires. Because some memory loss conditions can be progressive in nature, it is unknown how long an individual will continue to remember responses once practice has ended.

Booster sessions, or additional SR practices after the SR training has been discontinued, can be helpful for long-term retention if the information continues to be important for an individual (Cherry, Hawley, Jackson, & Boudreaux, 2009). Cherry et al. (2009) used SR to teach six people with dementia to associate a person's name with his or her face (face–name association). Three of the people were provided 6-, 12-, and 18-week booster sessions after SR practice ended. Six months later, the three people who had received the booster sessions recalled face–name associations more than the three people who did not receive the booster sessions. After the 6-month follow up, the three people who had not received the booster sessions were given additional SR practices and were able to re-establish the face–name associations in only a few days. This study established that conducting additional practice sessions within a few weeks or a few months of SR can help people with memory loss maintain the learned information for longer periods of time or help them to relearn the information if it is forgotten (Cherry, Hawley, Jackson, & Boudreaux, 2009). Hopper et al. (2010) found further support for using booster sessions to relearn forgotten information learned with SR. Examining the usefulness of SR when people with memory loss were trained to recall brand new information, these researchers found that previously known information is learned significantly faster than new information (Hopper, Drefs, Bayles, Tomoeda, & Dinu 2010).

Providing booster sessions is important because the needs and desires that have been addressed with SR likely remain relevant to the person. The purpose of SR is not to just teach people information to remember, but to help people learn and recall functional information to improve independence, safety, and quality of life. Checking in with the person with memory loss as well as other care partners is often the key to maintaining the positive outcomes achieved with SR. Healthcare professionals in long-term care settings are frequently required to conduct quarterly screenings of residents. These screenings can help evaluate retention and recall of information previously learned through SR. If these screenings reveal that memory loss has progressed to the point where the learned information is forgotten, booster treatment sessions can be introduced.

Summary

The SR procedure has been evolving through research and clinical application and has proven to be effective as a cognitive-training strategy. This chapter has provided a step-by-step guide for how to put SR into practice to address the needs and desires of people with memory loss. Before beginning SR, each care partner should complete a Spaced Retrieval Screening Form and Reading Screening Form to help lay a foundation for success for the individual with memory loss. The SR screening will determine if the individual is responsive to SR. The reading screening can assist in developing a continuous visual cue that can increase the likelihood of success during practice or an external memory aid to support memory following the discontinuation of the SR practice. Finally, long-term support of what has been taught is important if the information remains relevant. Refer to the Key Points and Practice Reminders for useful summary information regarding the SR process.

In Chapter 3, we introduce valuable tools that can be used to support SR, including visual cues, external memory aids, and modifications to the physical and social environment. We also discuss how various care team members can collaborate in implementing the SR strategy, increasing the likelihood of success for the person with memory loss.

KEY POINTS

Putting Spaced Retrieval into Practice

- Knowing the person well will help in determining his or her needs and desires.

- The lead question should be simple and direct. The person with cognitive impairment should be able to understand what is being asked.

- The lead question may need to be modified to increase success.

- The response may need to be modified to increase success.

- Practice intervals may need to be modified to eliminate incorrect responses.

- Build on success by increasing the length and difficulty of the response.

PRACTICE REMINDERS!

✓ Identify the need or desire.

✓ Develop the lead question.

✓ Formulate the response.

✓ Implement the practice intervals.

✓ Reinforce what was remembered.

Spaced Retrieval Screening Form

Name:_____ Date:_____

Lead Question:_____

Response: _____

Goal: *30 Seconds* _____

Practice Trial	Time Interval	Correct Response?			Notes
		Yes	No	NR	
1					
2					
3					
4					
5					
6					
7					
8					
9					
10					
11					
12					
13					
14					
15					

*NR=no response

Notes: _____

_____

_____

_____

_____

Spaced Retrieval Step by Step: An Evidence-Based Memory Intervention, by Jeanette E. Benigas, Jennifer A. Brush, and Gail M. Elliot. Copyright © 2016 by Health Professions Press, Inc. All rights reserved. www.healthpropress.com.

Reading Screening Form

Name: _____ Date: _____

Could the individual read before the onset of memory loss?

❑ Yes ❑ No

What language(s) does the individual read?

❑ English ❑ French

❑ Spanish ❑ Other _____

Does the individual require glasses?

❑ Yes ❑ No
  ❑ for distance
  ❑ for reading

Type size	Read the sentence aloud and do what it says.	Was the response read aloud?			For an incomplete response, circle which words were not read.	Was the task completed?		
		Yes	No	NR		Yes	No	NR
72 point	Pat your head.				Pat your head.			
48 point	Close your eyes.				Close your eyes.			
36 point	Point to the ceiling.				Point to the ceiling.			
24 point	Stick out your tongue.				Stick out your tongue.			
16 point	Touch your nose.				Touch your nose.			
12 point	Tap the table.				Tap the table.			

*NR=no response

Did the individual correctly read the name sign?

❑ Yes ❑ No ❑ No response

Did the individual correctly read the room number sign?

❑ Yes ❑ No ❑ No response

(continued)

Spaced Retrieval Step by Step: An Evidence-Based Memory Intervention, by Jeanette E. Benigas, Jennifer A. Brush, and Gail M. Elliot. Copyright © 2016 by Health Professions Press, Inc. All rights reserved. www.healthpropress.com.

Pat your head.

Close your eyes.

Point to the ceiling.

Stick out your tongue.

Touch your nose.

Tap the table.

Spaced Retrieval Step by Step: An Evidence-Based Memory Intervention, by Jeanette E. Benigas, Jennifer A. Brush, and Gail M. Elliot. Copyright © 2016 by Health Professions Press, Inc. All rights reserved. www.healthpropress.com.

Spaced Retrieval Data Form

Name: _____ Date: _____ Session Number: ____

Lead Question: _____

Response: _____

Did the person provide the correct response and perform the physical task correctly immediately following the lead question at first practice and without additional reinforcement and education?

❏ Yes   ❏ No   ❏ No response

Practice trial	Time interval	Continuous visual cue used?	Verbal response correct?			Physical task performed correctly?		
			Yes	No	NR	Yes	No	NR
1		❏ Y ❏ N						
2		❏ Y ❏ N						
3		❏ Y ❏ N						
4		❏ Y ❏ N						
5		❏ Y ❏ N						
6		❏ Y ❏ N						
7		❏ Y ❏ N						
8		❏ Y ❏ N						
9		❏ Y ❏ N						
10		❏ Y ❏ N						
11		❏ Y ❏ N						
12		❏ Y ❏ N						
13		❏ Y ❏ N						
14		❏ Y ❏ N						
15		❏ Y ❏ N						
16		❏ Y ❏ N						
17		❏ Y ❏ N						
18		❏ Y ❏ N						
19		❏ Y ❏ N						
20		❏ Y ❏ N						
21		❏ Y ❏ N						
22		❏ Y ❏ N						
23		❏ Y ❏ N						
24		❏ Y ❏ N						
25		❏ Y ❏ N						

Notes: _____

*NR=no response

Spaced Retrieval Step by Step: An Evidence-Based Memory Intervention, by Jeanette E. Benigas, Jennifer A. Brush, and Gail M. Elliot. Copyright © 2016 by Health Professions Press, Inc. All rights reserved. www.healthpropress.com.

CHAPTER 3

Beyond the Basics
Tools to Support Spaced Retrieval

Effective interventions for people with memory loss often involve making modifications to the physical and social environment in which a person lives (Brush, Calkins, Bruce, & Sanford, 2012). For example, simple changes to features in the environment that improve communication include modifying furnishings to create conversation areas (Bourgeois, 1991; Gottesman, 1965; Melin & Gotestam, 1981) or improving lighting and contrast so that conversation partners and needed items are more easily seen (Brush, Meehan, & Calkins, 2002). Other successful interventions incorporate verbal announcements and signs (Hanley, 1981; McClannahan & Risley, 1974); cue cards (Smith, 1988); diaries and watches (Hanley & Lusty, 1984); and memory notebooks and wallets (Bourgeois, 1992b; Mateer & Sohlberg, 1988).

This chapter discusses four physical, social, and environmental tools for supporting positive outcomes during Spaced Retrieval (SR) practice:

- continuous visual cues and external memory aids
- memory books
- wayfinding prompts
- involvement of all care team members

Guidelines are given for using each of these tools to enhance retention and recall of information.

Visual Cues and External Memory Aids

Visual cues and external memory aids can be combined with SR practice to facilitate learning and retention of information and physical tasks. A cue is a signal, situation, or piece of information that enhances a person's ability to retrieve details not recalled spontaneously. Cues that are placed in the physical environment can serve as helpful memory aids for all of us. For example, we rely on a variety of external memory aids in our day-to-day lives: lists to remember what to buy at the store, business cards to remember the name of someone recently met, pill organizers to stay on track with our medication, and road signs to point the way to our destination. Cues can also be tactile (i.e., items to touch and hold); olfactory (e.g., smelling burning toast); or auditory (e.g., hearing alarms). Enhancing cues in the physical and social environment helps persons with dementia successfully initiate and complete an activity by reducing demands on the impaired communication system and supporting pre-served abilities, such as through procedural memory (Brush et al., 2012) (see Chapter 1, this volume, for a complete description of procedural memory as well as other types of memory). For example, location and directional signs provide information so that a person no longer needs to ask for directions, which can be difficult for someone with communica-tion impairment. Cues such as picture sequencing cards or place setting templates make it easier for individuals to complete procedural memory tasks, such as dressing or setting the table. Cues can also be used to orient the person to time, place, and self, thus supporting the impaired episodic memory system. The Reading Screening Form (see Chapter 2) will help you get started in creating a continuous visual cue to support the SR practice or in choosing an external memory aid to use in the envi-ronment. The care partner can incorporate cues or external memory aids into SR training in a variety of ways:

- Use SR to help the person with memory loss to remember to use an external memory aid, such as a memory book, schedule, calendar, chore chart, diary, or sequencing card.

- Use an environmental cue to reinforce and maintain recall of the SR response. For example, placed by a favorite chair, an external memo-ry aid can prompt a person to perform a physical task correctly, such as remembering how to sit down properly. Care partners can support SR practice by using an external memory aid in the form of a cue card that says, "Reach for the arms of the chair before sitting."

- Use a continuous visual cue during all of the SR practices. The con-tinuous visual cue method involves placing the response to the lead question in writing in the person's line of sight during all of the SR practices, which supports both learning and retention (Benigas, 2013; Benigas & Bourgeois, in press). For example, a continuous visual cue can be placed on the table to help teach safe swallowing strategies (Benigas, 2013; Benigas & Bourgeois, in press; Brush & Camp, 1998b). The continuous visual cue provides the information about the compensatory swallow technique throughout the entire meal so that it continually reinforces the response that needs to be established. When the continuous visual cue is used, the environmental cue influences performance within and across sessions and supports the person's ability to remember for extended periods of time (Benigas, 2013; Benigas & Bourgeois, in press).

Implementing a Continuous Visual Cue During Spaced Retrieval

The following case example shows how a care partner can begin to use a continuous visual cue in SR.

 Meet Esther

Esther eats much too quickly, putting her at risk for choking. She enjoys eating a variety of foods while watching TV, including peanuts and popcorn. Esther lives in a long-term care community because she has dementia caused by Alzheimer's disease and can no longer care for herself at home safely. There is not enough staff for someone to sit with Esther at every meal and snack to remind her to eat slowly. The speech-language pathologist (SLP) has been asked to help reduce Esther's risk of choking so that she can safely snack and to maintain her quality of life. The following steps outline how to implement SR with Esther:

Five Easy Steps for Esther and the SLP

1. Esther's need: To remember to eat slowly.

2. The lead question the SLP will ask Esther: "What should you do when you eat?"

3. Esther's response will be: "Eat slowly."

4. The SLP will have Esther demonstrate eating slowly following every verbal response.

5. The SLP will help Esther to practice remembering to eat slowly using a continuous visual cue.

Eat slowly.

A continuous visual cue should have written on it the exact response the person is expected to give and is always in the person's line of sight.

The SLP scheduled the therapy sessions at the same time that Esther usually eats an afternoon snack. After completing the reading screening to assess Esther's reading ability (see Chapter 2), the SLP created a 3 × 5 notecard to place on the tabletop with the words "Eat slowly" in 28-point Calibri typeface. At the beginning of the session, before Esther ate any of her food, the SLP worked with Esther to practice remembering to eat slowly (see the dialogue exchange between the SLP and Esther).

> **SLP:** Esther, I would like you to enjoy your food safely. When you eat, it is important that you eat slowly. Here is a reminder for you. *(The SLP shows Esther a notecard with the words "Eat slowly" and then places the card directly above Esther's plate.)* Would you please show me how you eat slowly? *(Esther demonstrates for the SLP how she eats slowly.)* Great. You will be safe if you eat slowly. What should you do when you eat?
>
> **Esther:** Eat slowly.
>
> **SLP:** That is correct; please show me how you eat slowly.

While Esther ate her snack, the SLP implemented SR, increasing the time between practices using the recommended schedule (5 seconds [s], 10s, 20s, 30s, 1 minute [min], 2 min, 4 min, 8 min, and 16 min). After one week of sessions lasting 30–45 minutes using the continuous visual cue "Eat Slowly" and additional practice during snacks, Esther successfully recalled the information and demonstrated eating slowly at the first practice over three consecutive practice sessions. She also success-fully demonstrated eating slowly while dining independently outside of practice sessions. Next, the SLP updated the care plan to reflect the SR goals and the need for the continuous visual cue to always be in place whenever Esther eats.

The nursing and activity staff at the care community had already participated in an in-service about SR given by the SLP, so they were fa-miliar with the strategy. The SLP requested that the staff always set the continuous visual cue above Esther's plate for every meal and snack in-stead of at either side of the plate, to ensure she would see the reminder to eat slowly. Staff volunteered to check in with Esther throughout each meal and to help her practice remembering by asking, "What should you do when you eat?"

Memory Books

Memory books are external memory aids that have been widely used to enhance the conversational skills of people with dementia (Bourgeois, 1990, 1992a, 1992b). SR is an effective intervention for teaching people with memory loss to use external memory aids such as memory books (Bourgeois et al., 2003). When care partners use memory books, individu-als with memory loss have been shown to significantly increase the num-ber of factual statements; make more novel comments; and decrease the number of ambiguous, erroneous, and perseverative utterances through-out conversations (Bourgeois, 1990, 1992a, 1992b). By using memory books and communication aids, people with cognitive impairments have also displayed improved topic maintenance, increased length and num-ber of conversational turns, and decreased nonproductive utterances (Bourgeois, 1993; Bourgeois & Mason, 1996).

Memory books have a simple format. They should include one sim-ple photograph per page and underneath the photo should be one short phrase or declarative sentence that is relevant to the person with mem-ory loss. Embellishments and busy paper should be omitted (creating a memory book is different from creating a scrapbook). The books can include a schedule or routine for the day and text to help with orienta-tion, communication of needs, safety, reducing responsive behaviors, and increasing engagement in activities. When people with memory loss are unable to remember to use their memory book independently, SR can be a useful tool to help teach them when to use the book, how to use it, or where the memory book can be located in the living environment. (For detailed information about this important tool for supporting people with memory impairment, read *Memory and Communication Aids for People with Dementia* [Bourgeois, 2013].)

Using Spaced Retrieval to Support Wayfinding

Wayfinding is a process through which people use information in the environment to help them reach their desired destination. For those with memory loss conditions, the ability to independently reach destinations within the environment continues to be important in support of autonomy and quality of life (Marquardt & Schmieg, 2009). Often, spatial disorientation is among the very first symptoms to appear in Alzheimer's disease and becomes worse as the disease progresses (Alexander & Geschwind, 1984; Liu, Gauthier, & Gauthier, 1991; Richard & Bizzini, 1979). Poor wayfinding abilities in people with dementia

- affect safety (Rosswurm, Zimmerman, Schwartz-Fulton, & Norman, 1986)

- create conflict between residents (Rosswurm et al., 1986)

- cause unnecessary burden to long-term care staff (Everitt, Fields, Soumerai, & Avorn, 1991)

- cause anxiety, confusion, and panic (Passini, 2000)

- result in feelings of helplessness, raised blood pressure, headaches, increased physical exertion, and fatigue (Carpman & Grant, 2001)

- cause frustration, anger, or agitation (Zgola & Bordillon, 2001).

Care partners can use SR to support people with memory loss who need help with finding their way by teaching them to remember to look for cues in the environment. The most common forms of wayfinding cues are signs, landmarks, gestures, and verbal instructions. People with memory loss may require multiple types of environmental supports to achieve the greatest level of independence. Signage (pictures, words, or both) positioned strategically in the environment has proven to be an effective way to compensate for memory loss and help people reach their destinations (Bourgeois & Hickey, 2009; Brush, Camp, Bohach, & Gertsberg, 2015; Passini, Pigot, Rainville, & Tétreault, 2000). Although improvements in wayfinding for people with memory loss conditions such as dementia have been achieved without any intervention other than placing new signage in environments (Brush et al., 2015), others have found that signs alone have minimal effect on residents' orientation. McGilton et al.

(2003) questioned whether people with dementia could locate the dining room if they were provided with cues and shown how to find their way. While they could find their way 1 week after the intervention, this was not true 3 months later. These results suggest that ongoing repetition in the form of priming might improve performance over time. An earlier study found that the most important variable related to successful wayfinding cues was staff ensuring that residents were shown the sign and encouraged to use it (Hanley, 1981). While there is evidence to show that we need to compensate for this loss of wayfinding ability by putting the required information into the environment, the information alone is not always enough support. Once the information is in the environment, those who provide care have the responsibility to help the person with dementia use the memory aids. Care partners can use SR to remind the person about wayfinding cues and demonstrate how to use them (e.g., What do you look for when you have to use the toilet?). Wayfinding supports must be tailored for each individual and will differ as to where and how they are used. First, each environmental cue developed should be tested with the individual for whom it was designed. Environmental modifications include color, contrast, pictures, and landmarks to communicate information. The cue must be visible, familiar, understandable, clear (with no unnecessary markings), and in the user's line of sight.

Guidelines for Developing Visual Cues

The following sections present some guidelines and recommendations for developing visual cues.

Typography

Typographs are letters, numbers, words, or phrases used for communication. Consider the following when using typography in developing a visual cue:

- Begin by assessing whether the person was able to read prior to experiencing memory loss and make sure the person can still read before designing any written cue.

- To determine the type size that is easiest for the person to read, complete the Reading Screening Form described in Chapter 2. Begin with the sentence written in the largest type size and ask the person to read each line aloud and then do what it says. Ask the person to hold the page with the sentences in his or her nondominant hand and at a comfortable reading distance. Next, tape each sample sign one at a time to a wall at a height of 48–60 inches off the ground (use the lower height if the person is in a wheelchair), and ask the person to read each sentence while he or she is standing approximately 10–15 feet away. This test will help to determine the appropriate type size to use for signs.

- Use a sans serif typeface (U.S. Architectural and Transportation Barriers Compliance Board, n.d.; Vanderplas & Vanderplas, 1980). A sans serif typeface is one that does not have the small projecting hooks or tails called "serifs" at the end of strokes (*sans* means "without" in French). Examples of sans serif typeface include the fonts Arial, Calibri, Tahoma, and Helvetica.

- Use an uppercase letter at the beginning of a word followed by lowercase letters (e.g., Place, Sit). If writing a sentence, the first word should begin with an uppercase letter, and the rest of the words should begin with a lowercase letter. Avoid using text written in all capital letters, as studies have shown that people with dementia have a harder time processing text in all capitals (Dementia Services Development Centre, 2010; Hartley, 1994; Morrell & Echt, 1997).

<table>
<tr><td>

THIS IS HARDER
FOR SOMEONE
WITH DEMENTIA
TO READ.

</td><td>

This is easier
for someone
with dementia
to read.

</td></tr>
</table>

Color

When incorporating color into a visual cue, consider the following helpful tips:

- Color should be used in conjunction with other environmental cues, and the information being communicated through color should be consistent. For example, all dining room signs should be the same color.

- Predictability can be achieved in the environment through reliable repetition of key colors (Cohen & Weisman, 1991).

- Use room numbers and a distinguishing color for resident rooms and doors to enhance orientation (Lawton, Fulcomer, & Kleban, 1984).

- People older than 65 indicate a preference for blue, red, and green, in that order (Reeves, 1985; Van Wijk-Sijbesma, 2001). These colors can be used for landmarks or for sign backgrounds if the lettering is white.

- People with dementia indicate a preference for signs with a colored background with white letters more than signs with a white background (Brush et al., 2015).

- People with dementia tend to prefer signs with a background of bright green compared to dark green or white, bright magenta compared to dark purple or white, and bright royal blue compared to dark navy blue or white (Brush et al., 2015).

- To emphasize a sign, use brighter colors (using hue, value, and chroma) as well as a higher contrast with the background wall (Calkins, 2002).

Contrast

Contrast is the difference in luminance or color between objects. Contrast serves as a cue by helping people distinguish between different objects and helps to draw the attention of people who have difficulty staying on task or establishing orientation. When creating contrast, consider the following:

- Older people require as much as 300% more contrast than younger people for the recognition of objects in the environment (Tideiksaar, 1997).

- People with dementia present with significantly more impairment in contrast perception than cognitively intact older adults (Gilmore & Whitehouse, 1995).

- Increasing contrast in the environment can support functioning in people with dementia during such tasks as eating (Brush et al., 2002; Koss & Gilmore, 1998).

- Lack of environmental contrast can affect communication about care activities between care partners and people with dementia (Brush et al., 2012).

- There is evidence in the literature that the following color combinations work well in creating contrast: a brightly colored sign background with white letters, a black background with white letters, and a yellow background with black letters (Brush et al., 2012; Brush et al., 2015; Elliot, 2012). Test each combination with the individual for whom you are developing the visual cue and use the one that the person prefers.

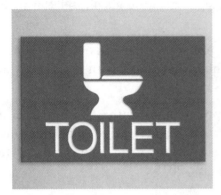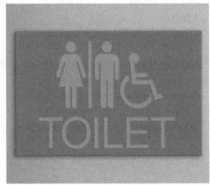

The sign on the left has high contrast and a pictograph that is easy to understand. The sign on the right has poor contrast and too many pictographs.

Pictographs

Pictographs are symbols representing people, places, or things. Use the following guidelines when incorporating a pictograph into a visual cue:

- Pictographs should contrast with the background of a sign and should be simple and easily understood by the person. Test several pictographs before choosing one to use on a visual cue.

- When using photographs of the person, make sure it is recognizable to him or her. Keep in mind that a person with memory loss may not recognize a picture from the present, but may easily identify a picture from the past.

- In a study comparing preferences for pictographs, people with dementia indicated a strong preference for the pictogram of a toilet over that of a pictogram of a male or female shape to indicate a restroom location (Brush et al., 2015).

Placement

When deciding where to place a visual cue, keep the following helpful tips in mind:

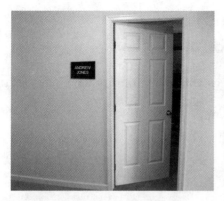 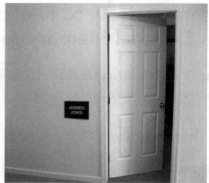

In comparison to the room sign on the right, the sign on the left may be placed too high for a person with dementia or someone who uses a wheelchair to see easily. The sign on the right is better positioned to be in the person's line of sight.

- Many older adults do not notice signs that are located on the upper sections of walls because they have limited range of motion in their upper body and walk looking at a level of 3 feet or lower (Brush et al., 2012; Passini, 2000).

- When people walk with a stooped posture, they may not see signs placed at the recommended height as advised by the U.S. Architectural and Transportation Barriers Compliance Board (n.d.).

- The Dementia Services Development Centre (2010) recommends that signs be mounted with their lower edge no higher than 4 feet from the floor. We recommend avoiding placement of signs on floors. It is important to encourage people to look up and see what is ahead of them in an effort to prevent falls.

Please note that this section is not a comprehensive guide for developing signage for your care community, but instead is meant to provide general guidelines and information for creating visual cues. The U.S. Architectural and Transportation Barriers Compliance Board (Access Board) provides guidelines in response to the Americans with Disabilities Act (1990) for the use of typographic signage in buildings for older adults. Guidelines recommend dark letters that contrast with a light background by at least 70%, sans serif fonts, no use of italics, tactile signs in uppercase letters (visual-only signs, such as directional signs, can be lowercase letters), and a mounting height of 60 inches (1,525 mm) above the floor to the centerline of the sign. Developing a wayfinding system is a complicated task that should be completed by someone with environmental design experience and knowledge of dementia care best practices.

Learning How to Find and Use an External Memory Aid

The following case example introduces you to one family who used SR to implement an external memory aid.

 Meet Sam

Sam is 23 years old and lives at home with his mother Alice and his father Bob. While growing up, he was very active in school and helped his parents around the house and in the yard. Because of a brain injury that he sustained in a car accident a year ago, Sam has a hard time becoming motivated in the mornings, and even if he is motivated, he cannot remember what he should do. As a result, Sam spends a lot of time sitting around and is starting to show signs of depression. The care team at the rehabilitation community where Sam stayed for several months worked with Alice to purchase a write-on/wipe-off whiteboard for the kitchen before Sam returned home. Alice hung the board next to the kitchen table, where it is easily in view when the family eats breakfast. Each morning, Alice writes two or three chores for Sam to do. She makes sure that these are tasks he would normally have completed prior to the accident and is able to safely accomplish now. Alice uses SR to help Sam remember to read the board each morning for his list of things to do. After he completes a chore, Alice walks back to the board with Sam and reminds him to cross it off the list. At the end of the day, Sam feels good that he has accomplished his chores. After Alice has helped Sam several times to remember to check his list of chores in the kitchen, he will begin to remember to do so on his own and will not need Alice's help anymore. Alice implemented the following five steps in using SR with Sam.

Five Easy Steps for Sam and Alice

1. Sam's need: To remember his household chores.

2. The lead question Alice will ask Sam: "Where do you look when you want to know what your chores are for the day?"

3. Sam's response will be (as he walks into the kitchen to read the whiteboard): "I check my list."

> ## Sam's Chores
> ___
> Laundry
>
> Take out trash
>
> Sweep leaves off
> the back deck

Write-on/wipe-off whiteboard hung next to the kitchen table with Sam's chores listed.

4. Alice will walk over to the whiteboard in the kitchen with Sam to make sure he sees and understands the information she has written for him.

5. Alice will help Sam to practice remembering to read the whiteboard (see the dialogue exchange between Alice and Sam).

Alice:	I would like to help you remember where you can look to find your chores for the day. You can check this list. *(Alice walks over to the whiteboard in the kitchen with Sam, shows him the list of chores written on it, and asks him to read the list.)* Sam, where do you look when you want to know what your chores are for the day?
Sam:	I check my list. *(Sam walks over to the whiteboard and reads the list of chores.)*
Alice:	That's right. We are going to keep trying to remember that. Sam, where do you look when you want to know what your chores are for the day?
Sam:	I have it written down some place.
Alice:	You can check your list right here. *(Alice shows Sam the whiteboard with the list written on it and then they both leave the kitchen. A few seconds pass.)* Sam, where do you look when you want to know what your chores are for the day?
Sam:	I check my list. *(Sam gives the correct response, but does not go into the kitchen and read the list from the whiteboard.)*
Alice:	That's right. Would you please show me your list? Or, let's go to the kitchen and check your list together.

Teaching Other Members of the Family and Care Team

A person's care team may include one family member or 10 healthcare professionals, depending on the setting and the person with whom you are working. If you provide home services, the care team might include a spouse, children, siblings, grandchildren, or friends. Family members have successfully implemented this strategy in the home setting (McKitrick & Camp, 1993). Since SR is easy to learn and implement, anyone can use it to help people with memory loss learn and remember in different care settings.

Once SR has been initiated with a person with memory loss and the person is having consistent success for a few days at recalling the information, the rest of the care team should be informed of the person's SR goals (remember that success at recalling information will be defined differently for different people.) In our clinical experience, SR works best when the entire care team works together to reinforce the information that has been taught and remembered. Therefore, once SR training has been established and the person is remembering the information for longer periods, it is time to teach others to ask the lead question, too. See the handout "Practice at Remembering: Information for the Care Team" at the end of the chapter for information on SR to share with anyone on the care team.

Before involving other members of the care team in the SR process, put the following guidelines into place to make the transition easier and more successful:

- Teach all members of the care team about SR and how it works.

- Discuss what the person's SR goals are at the care plan meeting, daily "stand up" meeting, or huddle.

- Document the SR goals in the care plan and as part of any information that is passed from staff to staff or staff to family.

- Create a quick and easy system for staff to record and communicate SR results, successes, and difficulties. Staff may choose to refer to the information from a chart stored on a computer, index cards in a box, or a notebook that is accessible to members of the care team. It is important to select a method of recording and communicating that fits into the existing structure and routines of the home setting or care center. You do not want to create additional work for staff. SR details should fit into existing communication strategies.

- Involve the family (with the person's consent) as much as possible. Visiting families are often pleased to practice SR because it gives them something meaningful to do and provides a significant way to be helpful.

Including the Care Team

The following case example shows how a care partner, Maria, includes other members of the care team in supporting the goals she is trying to accomplish in using SR with Luisa.

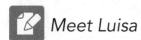 Meet Luisa

Luisa cannot remember that her husband Jorge visits every day at 2:00 p.m., so she often asks the nursing staff when he will be visiting. Luisa exhibits behaviors associated with anxiety when she is unsure if her husband will visit that day. Maria, who usually helps Luisa with her care routine, implements SR each morning during dressing and grooming using the recommended protocol.

Maria identified the following steps in working with Luisa:

1. Luisa's desire: To see her husband Jorge.

2. Luisa's need: To know what time Jorge is coming to visit, which will reduce her anxiety.

3. The lead question Maria will ask Luisa: "When time does Jorge come to visit?"

4. Luisa's response will be: "2:00"

5. Maria will practice with Luisa remembering when Jorge will come to visit her.

After one week of practicing each morning with Luisa, Maria asks the other staff on her shift to help Luisa practice remembering. She gives all members of the care team the handout "Practice at Remembering" and takes a few minutes to review the information with them. She teaches them to ask Luisa every once in a while the lead question (What time does Jorge come to visit?) and then wait for the response (2:00). In addition, Maria instructs the staff that if Luisa asks what time Jorge is coming to visit, they should tell her "2:00" and then immediately ask the lead question, "What time does Jorge come to visit?" This gives Luisa the information she is seeking while also giving her the opportunity to practice remembering it. At the change of shift, Maria explains the procedure to the next group of caregivers for Luisa's continued practice and reinforcement. The other staff do not have to follow the SR schedule of expanding intervals; Maria will continue to do so one-on-one with Luisa. The occasional practice that staff members give Luisa reinforces the work she is doing with Maria.

Keys to Success

When other members of the care team are involved in the SR process and tools such as visual cues are used, individuals with memory loss will experience greater independence because the supportive physical and social environment will enhance their recall of information. Keep the following keys to success in mind as you implement SR:

- Make the interaction meaningful to the person.
- Use the terminology and names for items that the person would commonly use.
- Be consistent with the lead question you ask.
- Be consistent with the response you accept as correct.
- Use SR to help the person with memory loss to remember to use an external memory aid (memory book, schedule, calendar, chore chart, diary, sequencing card).
- Use an environmental cue to reinforce and maintain recall of the SR response.
- Provide opportunities for practice throughout the day.
- If you cannot practice a number of times each day, practice when it is convenient.
- Practice one piece of information at a time.
- Involve the entire family or care team.
- Have fun!

Summary

This chapter has presented helpful tools for supporting SR and enhancing successful recall and retention of information in people with memory loss. Incorporating the use of continuous visual cues and external memory aids as well as making modifications to the physical and social environment can further assist a person with memory loss in wayfinding and communication. The entire care team should be involved in the SR process to reinforce the information learned and support the person's continued success. When prioritizing needs and desires or determining the best modifications to the SR practice, such as the timing of intervals, the care partner should use his or her best judgment in personalizing the approach to fit each individual. Ultimately, the best interest of the person being cared for is at the heart of SR.

Chapter 4 presents a variety of case examples of how SR can be used for people with memory loss. For each example, the SR strategy is customized to meet the unique need and desire of the individual as well as his or her rate of learning and success.

Practice at Remembering Information for the Care Team

Many people who are living with memory loss can learn and remember information, including facts and tasks. We can help individuals to learn and remember information by changing the way we teach the information. Telling someone the same thing repeatedly is not as effective as having the person practice at remembering the correct response.

Spaced Retrieval (SR) is a memory intervention that can be used to help a person with memory loss remember information over longer periods of time until the person can recall the information automatically. Care partners can use SR to give people with memory loss practice at remembering information until they can access it from memory with little cognitive effort. SR can be used to teach facts such as a date, room number, or phone number. It can also be used to help someone remember to take a medication, refer to a schedule, or complete a task. Correctly remembering information is rewarding for people with memory loss; episodes of forgetfulness are frustrating and can often be embarrassing. The objective in using SR is to create a learning opportunity that is successful.

Five Easy SR Implementation Steps for Care Partners:

1. Identify the need or desire.

2. Develop the lead question.

3. Formulate the response.

4. Implement the practice intervals.

5. Reinforce what was remembered.

When using SR, follow these five basic steps:

1. Begin by telling the person the information (the response), such as the following:
   - a phone number, address, or room number
   - the name of a loved one, neighbor, or care partner
   - the time that something routinely happens, such a taking medication or when a care partner arrives
   - a sign, landmark, or other cue for which to look when finding a destination

2. Ask the person the lead question.

3. Praise the person if the correct response was given.

(continued)

Spaced Retrieval Step by Step: An Evidence-Based Memory Intervention, by Jeanette E. Benigas, Jennifer A. Brush, and Gail M. Elliot. Copyright © 2016 by Health Professions Press, Inc. All rights reserved. www.healthpropress.com.

4. Provide the response right away if the lead question is answered incorrectly, or if there is a long pause indicating the person may be searching for the response, and then ask the lead question again immediately. Do not tell the person that he or she is wrong or made a mistake. Simply provide the correct response in a short and informative manner.

5. Increase the amount of time in between practices if the person answers correctly. Decrease the amount of time before asking the lead question again if the person answers incorrectly. Use the following recommended practice schedule:

Recommended Practice Schedule

5 seconds (s)→10s→20s→30s→1 minute (min)→2 min→4 min→8 min→16 min

Below are a few keys to success to keep in mind as you implement SR:

- Make the interaction meaningful to the person.
- Use the terminology and names for items that the person would commonly use.
- Be consistent with the lead question you ask.
- Be consistent with the response you accept as correct.
- Use SR to help the person with memory loss to remember to use an external memory aid (memory book, schedule, calendar, chore chart, diary, sequencing card).
- Use an environmental cue to reinforce and maintain recall of the SR response.
- Provide opportunities for practice throughout the day.
- If you cannot practice a number of times each day, practice when it is convenient.
- Practice one piece of information at a time.
- Involve the entire family or care team.
- Have fun!

Spaced Retrieval Step by Step: An Evidence-Based Memory Intervention, by Jeanette E. Benigas, Jennifer A. Brush, and Gail M. Elliot. Copyright © 2016 by Health Professions Press, Inc. All rights reserved. www.healthpropress.com.

Demonstrations of Spaced Retrieval

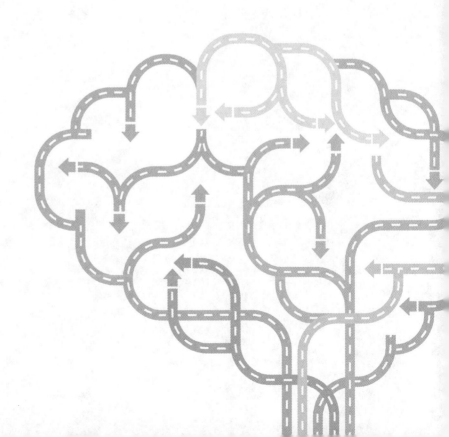

CHAPTER 4

Spaced Retrieval in Practice

Case Examples

This chapter includes case examples that illustrate the use of Spaced Retrieval (SR) in practice to address a diverse range of needs for people with memory loss. The cases feature either a professional or family care partner implementing SR. Each case outlines the step-by-step approach and includes examples of how to use the relevant forms presented in Chapter 2. Graphs that show the progress and outcomes of the SR practice are also included for each case.

Teaching a Multiple-Step Process

 Meet Mrs. Tech

Mrs. Tech has been diagnosed with early-stage Alzheimer's disease. She has been living on her own since her husband passed away less than a year ago. She is ambulatory but occasionally unsteady on her feet. Despite being unstable, she continues to do activities and chores around her home in the same way she did in the past. For example, she mentioned to her daughter Hilarie that she had climbed on a chair to take down her heavy curtains and then took them outside to air on the clothesline. She also frequently takes the bus to the mall when she wants to buy something rather than calling her daughter for a ride. Hilarie is concerned that her mother might fall while alone at home and may not be able to get help, or that she may get lost when she is in town. Mrs. Tech's daughter taught her to use a cell phone about 2 years ago so that she can contact someone if she needs assistance. Mrs. Tech used the cell phone periodically in the past, but she no longer remembers how to turn it on and has forgotten that it has to be charged regularly. Hilarie decided to reach out to the Here to Help Community Support Program to find out what she can do to help her mom. Liam, the occupational therapist at the Here to Help Program, came to visit Hilarie to discuss her mother's needs. Liam tells her about SR as a strategy to help her mother to remember important information (e.g., to charge, use, and keep her phone with her). He explains the process to Hilarie, namely that he will teach Mrs. Tech to charge, use, and keep her cell phone with her with the objective of keeping her as safe and independent as possible in her home and when she ventures out. See the Spaced Retrieval Screening Form that Liam used during his assessment of Mrs. Tech as well as a graph that shows the outcomes of the screening.

Spaced Retrieval Screening Form

Name: *Mrs. Tech*   Date: *January 21st*

Lead Question: *What is my name?*

Response: *Liam*

Goal: *30 Seconds*

Practice Trial	Time Interval	Correct Response?			Notes
		Yes	No	NR	
1	*5s*	*X*			
2	*10s*	*X*			
3	*20s*	*X*			
4	*30s*	*X*			*No difficulty noted*

NR=no response

Notes: *Mrs. Tech used her cell phone in the past. When asked where to press to turn on the phone she pointed to both the on and off buttons, but could not remember which one to press so she might be able to learn this skill quickly. She acquired the skill of using the phone in the past so this should make re-teaching the skill easier.*

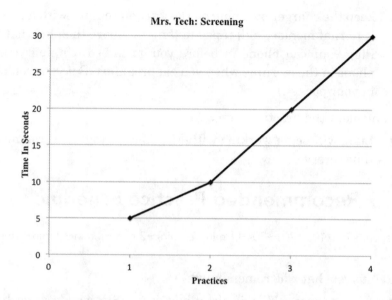

Six Easy Steps for Mrs. Tech and Her Daughter

1. Identify the desire:
   - Mrs. Tech desires to be independent but wants to be safe.

2. Identify the needs (each need should be addressed individually):
   - Mrs. Tech needs to learn how to use her cell phone.
   - Mrs. Tech needs to learn how to call a taxi when she wants to leave home or call Hilarie when she needs help.
   - Mrs. Tech needs to learn how to charge her cell phone, keep it with her, and use it when needed.

3. Develop the lead questions (each question should be addressed individually):
   - How do you turn on your cell phone?
   - What do you press to call a taxi and what do you press to call Hilarie?
   - How do you charge your cell phone?

4. Formulate the responses (each response should be addressed individually):
   - I press the button on top of the phone.
   - I press 1 for taxi and 2 for Hilarie.
   - I charge my cell phone in the kitchen before I go to bed, I unplug it when I eat breakfast, and I put it in my pocket. (Mrs. Tech will

keep the charger by a plug on the kitchen counter with a notecard [external memory aid] taped to the wall above the plug that says: Plug your cell phone in before you go to bed. Unplug your cell phone in the morning when you eat breakfast. Put your cell phone in your pocket.)

5. Implement the practice intervals:

   • Liam will begin working with Mrs. Tech using the recommended time interval:

Recommended Practice Schedule

5 seconds (s)→10s→20s→30s→1 minute (min)→2 min→4 min→8 min→16 min

---

6. Reinforce what was remembered:

   • Liam educates Hilarie about how to use SR to address each need individually.

   • Hilarie continues to work with her mother to reinforce the previously learned response for each individual need.

Identified Need #1

Liam begins to see Mrs. Tech and her daughter three times a week. During this time, Liam uses SR to teach Mrs. Tech how to turn on her cell phone and then educates Hilarie about how to use SR to address the other two needs that were identified. As they wait for each opportunity to practice, they all enjoy tea and cookies and look through photos in a family album. Liam teaches Hilarie to check the time on the clock in the room, so she pays special attention to where she sits before she begins to use SR with her mother. See the sample Spaced Retrieval Data Form that Liam used during his first session with Mrs. Tech as well as the graph showing session 1 outcomes.

Identified Need #2

After four sessions, Mrs. Tech successfully learns how to turn on her cell phone, as measured by the immediate recall at first practice over three consecutive sessions. Liam then begins to facilitate the SR practice between Mrs. Tech and Hilarie. He observes their interactions and provides feedback as needed. Liam decides that since Mrs. Tech learned how to turn on the cell phone so quickly, they would teach her to press 1

Spaced Retrieval Data Form

Name: *Mrs. Tech*   Date: *January 26th*   Session Number: *1*

Lead Question: *How do you turn on your cell phone?*

Response: *I press the button on top of the phone.*

Did the person provide the correct memory target immediately following the lead question at first practice without education?

❏ Yes   ☒ No   ❏ No response

Practice trial	Time interval	Continuous visual cue used?		Verbal response correct?			Physical task performed correctly?		
				Yes	No	NR	Yes	No	NR
1	5s	❏ Y	☒ N	X			X		
2	10s	❏ Y	☒ N	X			X		
3	20s	❏ Y	☒ N	X			X		
4	30s	❏ Y	☒ N	X			X		
5	1min	❏ Y	☒ N	X			X		
6	2min	❏ Y	☒ N	X			X		
7	4min	❏ Y	☒ N		X				X
8	2min	❏ Y	☒ N	X			X		
9	4min	❏ Y	☒ N	X			X		
10	8min	❏ Y	☒ N	X			X		

*NR=no response

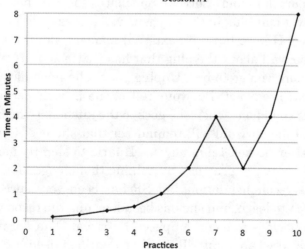

Mrs. Tech: How do you turn on your cell phone?
Session #1

for a taxi and 2 for Hilarie as part of the same response. If this becomes too difficult, Liam suggests that they could modify the approach by using two responses to two different lead questions. In other words, they would just focus on teaching Mrs. Tech to call the taxi, and once she learned to press 1, they would then teach her to press 2 for her daughter as a second response. Liam records the outcomes during their sessions together, but Hilarie expresses to him that she does not plan to use the Spaced Retrieval Data Form when she works with her mother on her own. During the second session, Mrs. Tech has very little difficulty learning the combined response of pressing 1 for a taxi and pressing 2 to reach her daughter. Liam determines that it would be acceptable to continue to use the combined response in future practice sessions. See the Spaced Retrieval Data Form that Liam used during the second session and a graph showing the outcomes for the second identified need.

Hilarie continues to work with her mother to reinforce the previously learned response by asking her lead question #1, How do you turn on your cell phone? After Mrs. Tech answers with the correct response, her daughter then follows with the second target question, What do you press to call a taxi and what do you press to call Hilarie? During this time, Liam begins to consult with Mrs. Tech's daughter through a weekly phone call.

Identified Need #3

Once Mrs. Tech learns to use her cell phone to dial a taxi and her daughter, which was measured by immediate recall at first practice over three consecutive sessions, Hilarie then uses SR to teach her mother to charge her cell phone. This time, before initiating SR, Hilarie modifies the environment to support her mom's success. She places the cell phone charger by the most convenient plug in the kitchen, which is easy for her mother to access and see. Hilarie tapes an external memory aid in the form of a notecard to the wall above the plug that has written on it: "Plug your cell phone in before you go to bed. Unplug your cell phone in the morning when you eat breakfast. Put your cell phone in your pocket." Mrs. Tech will see the cell phone when she goes to the kitchen in the morning, and the external memory aid will remind her that she needs to unplug it and put it in her pocket. Liam advises Hilarie to slightly modify the time intervals in between practices by making them longer. He does not often make this recommendation, but SR has been very successful in helping Mrs. Tech to learn, and she has been learning the responses very quickly. Hilarie decides to use the Spaced Retrieval Data Form to help keep her organized when using SR for this identified need because she is adding in an external memory aid and increasing the time intervals.

Spaced Retrieval Data Form

Name: *Mrs. Tech*   Date: *February 6th*   Session Number: *6*

Lead Question: *What do you press to call a taxi and what do you press to call your daughter?*

Response: *1 for taxi and 2 for Hilarie*

Did the person provide the correct memory target immediately following the lead question at first practice without education?

☒ Yes   ❏ No   ❏ No response

Practice trial	Time interval	Continuous visual cue used?		Verbal response correct?			Physical task performed correctly?		
				Yes	No	NR	Yes	No	NR
1	5s	❏ Y	☒ N	X			X		
2	10s	❏ Y	☒ N	X			X		
3	20s	❏ Y	☒ N	X			X		
4	30s	❏ Y	☒ N	X			X		
5	1min	❏ Y	☒ N	X			X		
6	2min	❏ Y	☒ N	X			X		
7	4min	❏ Y	☒ N		X				X
8	2min	❏ Y	☒ N	X			X		
9	4min	❏ Y	☒ N	X			X		
10	8min	❏ Y	☒ N		X		X		X
9	4min	❏ Y	☒ N	X			X		
10	8min	❏ Y	☒ N	X			X		

*NR=no response

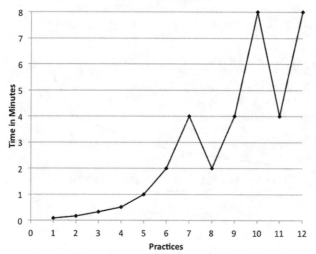

Mrs. Tech: 1 for taxi and 2 for Hilarie
Session #6

Spaced Retrieval Data Form

Name: *Mrs. Tech*   Date: *February 13th*   Session Number: *9*

Lead Question: *How do you charge your phone?*

Response: *I charge my phone in the kitchen before bed, unplug it when I eat breakfast and put it in my pocket.*

Did the person provide the correct memory target immediately following the lead question at first practice without education?

❑ Yes   ☒ No   ❑ No response

Practice trial	Time interval	Continuous visual cue used?		Verbal response correct?			Physical task performed correctly?		
				Yes	No	NR	Yes	No	NR
1	10s	☒ Y	❑ N	X			X		
2	30s	☒ Y	❑ N	X			X		
3	1min	☒ Y	❑ N	X			X		
4	2min	☒ Y	❑ N	X			X		
5	7min	☒ Y	❑ N	X			X		

*NR=no response

Notes: *Mom got tired during this session, so we will practice more tomorrow.*

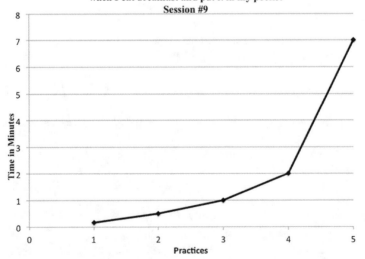

Mrs. Tech: I charge my phone in the kitchen before bed, unplug it when I eat breakfast and put it in my pocket
Session #9

Hilarie implements the SR practice with her mother in the kitchen and she places the external memory aid in Mrs. Tech's line of sight. This way, Mrs. Tech can learn and practice the physical task of plugging in her cell phone, unplugging it, and putting it in her pocket at the actual location where she will be expected to perform the routine on a daily basis. See the Spaced Retrieval Data Form that Hilarie used and a graph showing the outcomes during the first session for the third identified need.

After three more practice sessions, Hilarie calls Liam and tells him that her mother has been able to learn the two-step approach quickly. She also says that her mom used the external memory aid, so she will keep it taped above the plug as a reminder to charge the cell phone.

One month later, Mrs. Tech is doing well. She continues to keep her cell phone with her, which makes communication with her daughter easier. She occasionally forgets to charge the cell phone, but remembers how to call the taxi and her daughter. Hilarie decides to continue to use SR to help her mom maintain her independence and safety. She is now teaching her to dial 911 if she falls and is unable to get up.

Teaching New Habits Over Old Ones

 Meet Mr. Farmer

Mr. Farmer spent his life living and working on his family farm. He loved working in the fields and still talks about how much he enjoyed the time he spent with the farm animals. Mr. Farmer, who has been widowed for 3 years, is a friendly, quiet man who now lives in a long-term care community. He suffered a stroke 4 years ago, and although he has regained a lot of function, he has difficulty with his memory. Mr. Farmer lived independently for several months after his stroke, but could not manage on his own after his wife passed away, so arrangements were made to move him to a long-term care community. His ambulation is good, and he often walks throughout the halls. Occasionally, however, he stops to urinate on the walls. This upsets the staff and residents. While Mr. Farmer is a very pleasant man, the other residents say unkind words about him and make it clear they want nothing to do with him. Mr. Farmer is saddened when he hears people's negative comments. He does not understand why they are acting this way toward him. He does not remember or realize that he has been urinating on walls and not in the bathroom. Persons with memory loss often lack the insight that would help them connect their actions and the respective consequences.

When Bea, the Director of Care, considered why he might be urinating on the walls, she recalls that earlier in life he was used to going to the bathroom in the open fields while working on his family farm. Therefore, this behavior became habitual and automatic for Mr. Farmer; he did not have the habit of returning to the farmhouse to use the toilet. As mentioned in Chapter 1, habits are part of nondeclarative or procedural memory, which is often spared with memory loss. Bea helps the staff to understand that when Mr. Farmer urinates on the walls, he has forgotten that he lives in a long-term care community and is simply doing what he always did. The behavior is not intentional.

Bea needs to help change Mr. Farmer's habit by helping him to remember to find and use the toilet. Before she begins, she needs to find out which toileting words are meaningful and familiar to him. She knows that residents use many different words related to toileting, such as washroom, restroom, toilet, commode, men's room, can, water closet, and urinal. She has learned that some of the words, such as *washroom*, are often misunderstood, as someone with memory loss may take the term literally and relate the word *washroom* with having a bath or getting washed. Bea's objective is to use a word that is relevant and concrete to Mr. Farmer (see dialogue exchange between Bea and Mr. Farmer). The word *toilet* represents a physical object, so she wants to use this word as much as possible. Since people go to a toilet to relieve themselves, the word *toilet* reinforces the appropriate place for urination. Bea begins by completing the Spaced Retrieval Screening and Reading Screening forms with Mr. Farmer to confirm that her plan to implement an SR process would be suitable for him (see Mr. Farmer's Reading Screening Form).

Bea:	Mr. Farmer, when you have to go to the toilet, what do you say? Do you say, "I have to go to the bathroom," "I have to go to the toilet," or do say use a different phrase?
Mr. Farmer:	I don't know (*paired with a shrug of his shoulders*).
Bea:	Would it be okay to use the phrase "go to the toilet"?

Reading Screening Form

Name: *Mr. Farmer*   Date: *April 10th*

Could the individual read before the onset of memory loss?

☒ Yes   ☐ No

What language(s) does the individual read?

☒ English   ☐ French

☐ Spanish   ☐ Other _____

Does the individual require glasses?

☐ Yes   ☒ No
  ☐ for distance
  ☐ for reading

Type size	Read the sentence aloud and do what it says.	Was the response read aloud?			For an incomplete response, circle which words were not read.	Was the task completed?		
		Yes	No	NR		Yes	No	NR
72 point	Pat your head.	✗			Pat your head.	✗		
48 point	Close your eyes.	✗			Close your eyes.	✗		
36 point	Point to the ceiling.	✗			Point to the ceiling.	✗		
24 point	Stick out your tongue.	✗			Stick out your tongue.	✗		
16 point	Touch your nose.		✗		(Touch) your (nose.)	✗		
12 point	Tap the table.			✗	Tap the table.			✗

Six Easy Steps for Mr. Farmer and Bea

1. Identify the desire:
   - Mr. Farmer desires to have friends and to stop the unkind words and behaviors of fellow residents.

2. Identify the needs:
   - Mr. Farmer needs to know where the toilet is.
   - Mr. Farmer needs to use the toilet and not the wall when urinating.

3. Develop the lead question:
   - What do you do when you need to use the toilet?

4. Formulate the response:
   - Follow the arrow to the toilet. (Bea will teach Mr. Farmer to point to the arrow labeled "to toilet" and to follow it to the toilet sign on the bathroom door.)

5. Implement the practice intervals:
   - Bea will begin working with Mr. Farmer using the recommended time interval:

Recommended Practice Schedule

5 seconds (s)→10s→20s→30s→1 minute (min)→2 min→4 min→8 min→16 min

---

6. Reinforce what was learned:
   - Other staff will ask Mr. Farmer the lead question at least a few times a day to ensure he remembers to follow the arrow to the toilet sign on the bathroom door when he needs to urinate.

Before Bea begins to teach Mr. Farmer what he needs to do, she modifies the environment by posting a sign on the wall directly outside his bedroom door. The sign has an arrow pointing to his room underneath the word *toilet*. The sign is written in large, bold letters using a 24-point sans serif typeface. Bea also places a picture of a toilet on the door of his bathroom inside his bedroom. Finally, Bea puts black tape on the toilet seat to make sure Mr. Farmer can clearly see where to aim when urinating and she also puts in a request to purchase a colored toilet seat. She does this because the toilet seat and the floor are both white, which makes the target area difficult for Mr. Farmer to see.

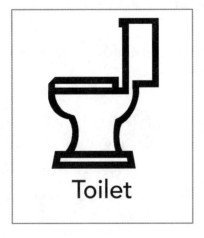
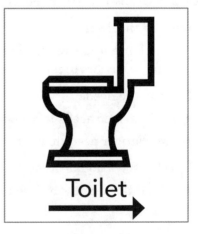

Bea then implements the first practice session with Mr. Farmer (see the dialogue exchange between Bea and Mr. Farmer).

She asks Mr. Farmer the lead question, waits for him to provide the response, and then prompts him to perform the physical task of finding the arrow and following it to the bathroom. Bea continues to practice with Mr. Farmer while standing in front of the arrow and asks him to point to it following each response until the time intervals are long enough for Mr. Farmer to start walking from the arrow to the bathroom door after he gives his response. This will give Mr. Farmer repeated practice in both recalling the correct information and remembering to read the sign and then walk to the bathroom until the old habit of urinating on the walls becomes a new habit of instead using the toilet. (See the Spaced Retrieval Data Form and a graph showing the outcomes during the fifth practice session for Mr. Farmer.)

After seven SR practice sessions, Mr. Farmer stops urinating on the walls. Bea asks staff to reinforce these positive outcomes by asking Mr. Farmer the lead question at least a few times a day to ensure the new habit does not change. The staff connects him with residents by inviting him to participate in a variety of activities. The other residents soon for-

Bea:	Today we're going to practice finding the toilet. When you need to use the toilet, follow the arrow. What do you do when you need to use the toilet? *(Bea is standing right in front of the arrow so Mr. Farmer can see it. She expects an immediate response to the lead question.)*
Mr. Farmer:	Follow the arrow to the toilet.
Bea:	Yes, that's right. Follow the arrow to the toilet. We're going to keep trying to remember that. Please show me the arrow. *(Mr. Farmer points to the arrow.)* (5-second delay) Mr. Farmer, what do you do when you need to use the toilet?
Mr. Farmer:	Follow the arrow to the toilet. *(He points to the arrow as he speaks.)*
Bea:	That's right. Let's see if you can remember for longer this time. *(10-second delay)* Mr. Farmer, what do you do when you need to use the toilet?
Mr. Farmer:	Follow the arrow to the toilet. *(He points to the arrow after he gives the response.)*
Bea:	That's right.

Spaced Retrieval Data Form

Name: *Mr. Farmer*   Date: *April 17th*   Session Number: *5*

Lead Question: *What do you do when you need to use the toilet?*

Response: *Follow the arrow to the toilet.*

Did the person provide the correct memory target immediately following the lead question at first practice without education?

☒ Yes   ❑ No   ❑ No response

Practice trial	Time interval	Continuous visual cue used?	Verbal response correct?			Physical task performed correctly?		
			Yes	No	NR	Yes	No	NR
1	5s	☒Y ❑N	X			X		
2	10s	☒Y ❑N	X			X		
3	20s	☒Y ❑N	X			X		
4	30s	☒Y ❑N	X			X		
5	1min	☒Y ❑N	X			X		
6	2min	☒Y ❑N	X			X		
7	4min	☒Y ❑N	X			X		
8	8min	☒Y ❑N	X			X		
9	16min	❑Y ☒N		X			X	
10	8min	❑Y ☒N		X				X
11	4min	☒Y ❑N	X			X		
12	8min	☒Y ❑N	X			X		
13	16min	☒Y ❑N	X			X		

*NR=no response

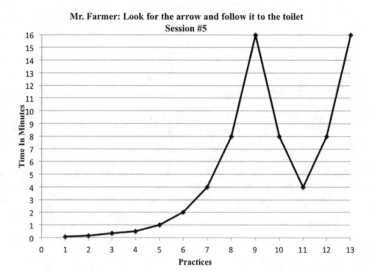

Mr. Farmer: Look for the arrow and follow it to the toilet
Session #5

get that he had urinated on the walls. They no longer shun him and stop the unkind words. Mr. Farmer appears to be a much happier person since learning to use the toilet and not the wall when urinating.

Some might wonder if a toilet sign on the wall outside of a resident's room would be confusing for other residents. Bea determined she would use an external memory aid as part of the SR practice with Mr. Farmer after considering his needs as well as the possible outcomes that may result from placing it in the hall versus just in his room. Since Mr. Farmer was urinating on the walls, she decided it had to be put outside of his room. The unit Mr. Farmer lives on is small and he rarely uses the public bathroom. Bea, therefore, determined it was best to teach Mr. Farmer the appropriate act of urinating in the toilet where he goes most often (his room), and not where he might go.

Adapting the Strategy When Progress Is Slow

 Meet Jack

Jack has been living in a long-term care community for just over a month. His family convinced him to move to a place where there was more to do each day and where people could help him with meals and laundry. He did not like cooking and recognized that he was having trouble managing and remembering things, so he agreed to move. Jack did not know if he would like living at a long-term care community, but a friend lives there too, and so he settled in fairly well. Jack has Parkinson's disease and is unsteady on his feet. He needs to use a walker, but often forgets and has had several recent falls. He also struggles to remember where he is and constantly tells people he needs to go home. He wanders into other people's rooms regularly and always says that he is trying to head home or that he is looking for his room. When people remind him that he lives at the Enjoying Life Home, he says, "Oh, I forgot." The staff begin to think about Jack's needs and consider that he may need to use a wheelchair with an alarm to prevent him from falling, but are reluctant because they know it would take away some of his independence. The care community doctor refers Jack to Stephanie, the speech-language pathologist, who will use SR to teach him to remember where he lives and to use his walker to prevent him from falling.

Six Easy Steps for Jack and Stephanie

1. Identify the desire (each desire should be addressed individually):
   - Jack desires to avoid falling.
   - Jack desires to stop forgetting where he lives.

2. Identify the needs:
   - Jack needs to remember to use his walker.
   - Jack needs to remember that he lives at the Enjoying Life Home.

3. Develop the lead questions (each question should be addressed individually):
   - What should you use every time you walk?
   - Where do you live?

4. Formulate the responses (each response should be addressed individually):
   - My walker
   - Enjoying Life Home

5. Implement the practice intervals:
   - Stephanie will begin working with Jack using the recommended time interval:

Recommended Practice Schedule

5 seconds (s)→10s→20s→30s→**1 minute (min)**→2 min→4 min→8 min→16 min

---

6. Reinforce what was learned:
   - Other staff members reinforce the practice by asking Jack what he should use every time he walks.

Stephanie begins by conducting a clinical evaluation, which includes a cognition screening as well as both the SR and reading screenings. Jack has some difficulty during the SR screening, which surprises Stephanie because he is very talkative and responsive to questions. At the end of her evaluation, Stephanie determines that although Jack's cognitive

Spaced Retrieval Screening Form

Name: *Jack*   Date: *August 1st*

Lead Question: *What is my name?*

Response: *Stephanie*

Goal: *30 Seconds*

Practice Trial	Time Interval	Correct Response?			Notes
		Yes	No	NR	
1	5s	X			
2	10s		X		
3	5s	X			
4	10s	X			
5	20s		X		
6	10s		X		
7	5s		X		
8	10s	X			
9	20s	X			
10	30s	X			

NR=no response

Notes: *Jack mentioned at the end of the session he has never been good with names.*

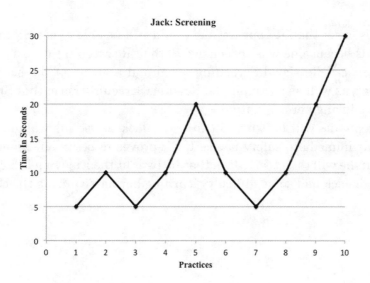

Jack: Screening

Reading Screening Form

Name: *Jack*   Date: *August 1st*

Could the individual read before the onset of memory loss?

☒ Yes   ❑ No

What language(s) does the individual read?

☒ English   ❑ French

❑ Spanish   ❑ Other _____

Does the individual require glasses?

☒ Yes   ❑ No

   ❑ for distance
   ☒ for reading

Type size	Read the sentence aloud and do what it says.	Was the response read aloud?			For an incomplete response, circle which words were not read.	Was the task completed?		
		Yes	No	NR		Yes	No	NR
72 point	Pat your head.	✗			Pat your head.	✗		
48 point	Close your eyes.	✗			Close your eyes.	✗		
36 point	Point to the ceiling.	✗			Point to the ceiling.	✗		
24 point	Stick out your tongue.	✗			Stick out your tongue.	✗		
16 point	Touch your nose.	✗			Touch your nose.	✗		
12 point	Tap the table.		✗		Tap the (table.)			✗

ability is lower than it appears, she would still be able to use SR to meet his needs because he was responsive to the SR screening. (See a sample of the Spaced Retrieval Screening Form and a graph of the screening outcomes, as well as a sample the Reading Screening Form that Stephanie used during her evaluation.)

Stephanie will first use SR to teach Jack to use his walker to address his immediate safety needs. If SR proves to be an effective intervention, she will then teach Jack that he lives at the Enjoying Life Home. Although Jack had some difficulty learning her name during the clinical evaluation, Stephanie determines that she will follow the recommended SR protocol without any modifications unless she finds they are needed.

Before she begins the practice, Stephanie creates a continuous visual cue using a white piece of 8.5 × 11.5 paper with the expected target response, "my walker," printed in a 16-point sans serif typeface. She folds the piece of paper in half like a tent and places it in front of Jack during practice. She also makes sure Jack has his reading glasses for each session. For the first practice, Jack is unable to recall the response for more than 30 seconds. After Jack could not remember the response for 1 minute after three consecutive attempts, Stephanie stops for the day. She is unsure if Jack will have successful outcomes, but she decides to try again after two days. For the next session, Jack is more responsive to the practice, but his progress is slow. Stephanie then meets with the staff at Enjoying Life Home and educates them about the SR strategy, including providing them with the handout Practice at Remembering: Information for the Care Team (see Chapter 3). She tells them she is teaching Jack to remember to use his walker during all ambulation. She also tells them that if the practice is successful, she will then teach Jack that he lives at Enjoying Life Home. She asks them to help her to reinforce the practice by asking Jack what he should use every time he walks. She explains that implementing the SR approach will work best if Jack is given the opportunity to practice remembering multiple times throughout the day. The staff agree to work with Jack to reinforce his learning. (See the Spaced Retrieval Data Form that Stephanie prepared for the third session and a graph of the outcomes.)

Although Jack is doing better, he is very inconsistent with remembering the response immediately at the beginning of each session. After 15 practice sessions, Jack remembers to use his walker whenever he ambulates. Stephanie determines that she will continue using SR to teach Jack where he lives. However, instead of doubling the time intervals, she shortens them to help increase Jack's success in providing the correct response. She uses the following modified time intervals:

5 seconds (s)→10s→20s→30s→1 minute (min)→1 minute (min)→2 min→4 min→7 min→11 min

Stephanie keeps the scientific principle of the spacing effect in mind, remembering to make sure the intervals continue to increase instead of being equal. The modified procedure proves successful. Jack learns that he lives at Enjoying Life Home after 10 sessions.

Spaced Retrieval Data Form

Name: Jack   Date: August 12th   Session Number: 3

Lead Question: What should you use every time you walk?

Response: My walker.

Did the person provide the correct memory target immediately following the lead question at first practice without education?

☑ Yes   ☐ No   ☐ No response

Practice trial	Time interval	Continuous visual cue used?	Verbal response correct?			Physical task performed correctly?		
			Yes	No	NR	Yes	No	NR
1	5s	☐ Y ☑ N	X			X		
2	10s	☐ Y ☑ N	X			X		
3	20s	☑ Y ☐ N	X			X		
4	30s	☑ Y ☐ N	X			X		
5	1min	☑ Y ☐ N	X			X		
6	2min	☐ Y ☑ N		X				X
7	1min	☑ Y ☐ N	X				X	
8	2min	☐ Y ☑ N		X			X	
9	1min	☑ Y ☐ N	X			X		
10	2min	☑ Y ☐ N	X			X		
11	4min	☑ Y ☐ N	X			X		
12	8min	☑ Y ☐ N	X			X		
13	16min	☑ Y ☐ N	X			X		

*NR=no response

Notes: Sometimes Jack needs a verbal cue to look at the card so he can remember.

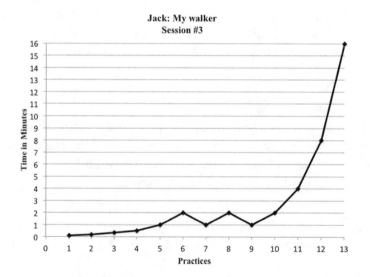

Jack: My walker
Session #3

Ensuring Safety with a Daily Activity

 Meet Betty

Betty lives in a one-story home with her daughter, son-in-law, and two grandchildren. She recently had a hip replacement and is staying at a post-acute rehabilitation center for physical therapy before she returns home. Betty has not been diagnosed with any conditions that could result in memory loss and has never been forgetful, but she seems to be having some trouble with her memory since her surgery. She is making great gains with her walking, but the physical therapist, Richard, has noticed that her sit-to-stand transfer sequencing is unsafe. Betty needs to use a walker following her surgery, and when standing up she often grabs for the walker first, which is on wheels. Richard has decided to use SR to teach Betty how to stand up safely while he facilitates her exercises in the therapy room.

Six Easy Steps for Betty and Richard

1. Identify the desire:
   - Betty desires to be able to stand up safely.

2. Identify the need:
   - Betty needs to learn how to stand up safely.

3. Develop the lead question:
   - How do you stand up safely?

4. Formulate the response:
   - I put my hands on the chair or bed, push up, and then step inside the walker.

5. Implement the practice intervals:
    - Richard will begin working with Betty using the recommended time interval:

Recommended Practice Schedule

5 seconds (s)→10s→20s→30s→**1 minute (min)**→2 min→4 min→8 min→16 min

---

6. Reinforce what was remembered:
    - Richard also teaches Katie, Betty's granddaughter, how to reinforce helping her grandmother to remember how to stand up safely.

Richard begins by assessing Betty using the Spaced Retrieval Screening Form. He chooses not to administer the reading screening because Betty regularly reads the morning newspaper and then discusses the daily news with the therapists, indicating that she can read a small type size and comprehend what she had read. (See the sample of the Spaced Retrieval Screening Form and a graph showing the screening outcomes.)

As a former elementary school teacher, Betty expresses to Richard how important it is to her to be able to practice and learn how to stand up safely for when she returns home. Her 14-year-old granddaughter, Katie, visits her after school each day, so Richard waits to give Betty her first SR practice until Katie arrives. During the first session, Richard provides Katie with the Practice at Remembering handout (see Chapter 3) and educates her about the SR protocol. He teaches both Betty and Katie how the physical act of standing up safely should be properly performed, has them practice several times to demonstrate their understanding, and stresses how important it is to have Betty perform standing up safely immediately following each correct response to the lead question (see the dialogue exchange between Richard and Betty). Richard creates two identical continuous visual cues, one to keep in the treatment room and a second to give to Betty and Katie to use during their one-on-one practices. The continuous visual cues state the target response: I put my hands on the chair or bed, push up, and then step inside the walker. They are printed on two white 8.5 × 11.5 pieces of paper in a 12-point sans serif typeface and folded in half like a tent. Throughout the session, Katie observes and eagerly takes notes. (See the sample Spaced Retrieval Data Form that Richard asked Katie to use and a graph showing the outcomes of the second session.)

Spaced Retrieval Screening Form

Name: *Betty*   Date: *November 6th*

Lead Question: *What is my name?*

Response: *Richard*

Goal: *30 Seconds*

Practice Trial	Time Interval	Correct Response?			Notes
		Yes	No	NR	
1	5s	x			
2	10s	x			
3	20s	x			
4	30s	x			

NR=no response

Notes: *Betty is a former elementary school teacher and is highly motivated to learn her strategy. She would like to have therapy in the afternoon when her granddaughter is visiting, so they can practice together in the evenings and over the telephone.*

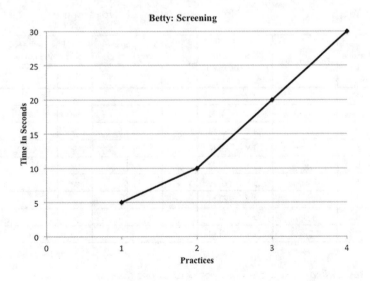

> *Richard:* Betty, how do you stand up safely?
>
> *Betty:* I put my hands on the chair or bed, push up, and then step inside the walker.
>
> *Richard:* Good! Please show me how to stand up safely. *(Betty demonstrates the physical task of standing up.) (16-minute delay; time interval is filled with exercises to address other goals)* Betty, how do you stand up safely?
>
> *Betty:* I put my hands on the chair or bed, push up, and then step inside the walker. *(Betty stands up immediately after giving the response.)*

Spaced Retrieval Data Form

Name: *Betty*　　　　Date: *November 7th*　　Session Number: *2*

Lead Question: *How do you stand up safely?*

Response: *I put my hands on the chair or bed, push up, and then step inside the walker.*

Did the person provide the correct memory target immediately following the lead question at first practice without education?

☒ Yes　　　　　❑ No　　　　　❑ No response

Practice trial	Time interval	Continuous visual cue used?		Verbal response correct?			Physical task performed correctly?		
				Yes	No	NR	Yes	No	NR
1	5s	❑ Y	☒ N	X			X		
2	10s	❑ Y	☒ N	X			X		
3	20s	❑ Y	☒ N	X			X		
4	30s	❑ Y	☒ N	X			X		
5	1min	❑ Y	☒ N	X			X		
6	2min	❑ Y	☒ N	X			X		
7	4min	❑ Y	☒ N	X			X		
8	8min	❑ Y	☒ N	X			X		
9	16min	❑ Y	☒ N	X			X		

*NR=no response

Notes: *Grandma said she does not need to use the sign.*

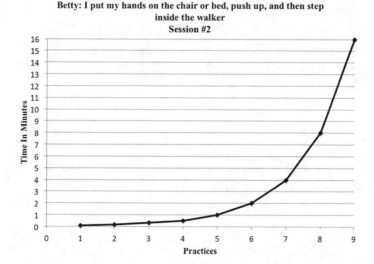

Betty: I put my hands on the chair or bed, push up, and then step inside the walker
Session #2

As SR practice sessions continue, Betty finds that it is often helpful for her to say the response to the lead question while demonstrating the physical task at the same time. She rarely provides an incorrect response, so Richard is fine with her decision to give the response while standing safely.

Betty is able to learn how to stand up safely after four sessions and returns home shortly thereafter. Once home, she finds that she still has some mild difficulty with her memory and begins to use SR with Katie to help her to remember to take her afternoon pills.

Summary

The case examples presented in this chapter demonstrate how to implement SR in a variety of settings. The examples illustrate the importance of personalizing this strategy based on the individual as well as the need to collaborate with all members of the care team to maximize success. The concluding chapter of the book provides an overview of the extensive body of research supporting SR and touches on the future of this intervention.

Research Behind Spaced Retrieval

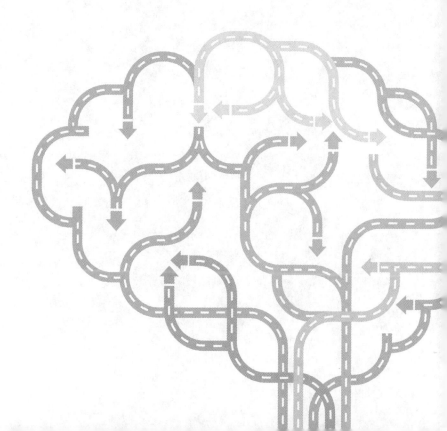

CHAPTER 5

Spaced Retrieval Snapshot

This book has outlined a step-by-step approach to implementing SR that any care partner can put into practice. The strategy has strengthened over time through thoughtful development by clinicians and researchers seeking to improve quality of life for those with dementia. Further, evidence now shows its effectiveness for a variety of other memory loss conditions. Due to the extensive research available, which this chapter reviews, the strategy is very flexible.

More than two decades of research and clinical practice have contributed to the SR strategy as it exists today. This chapter summarizes published research on SR and a selection of published articles related to the spacing effect, expanded retrieval, and errorless learning available at the time of this book's publication. This review includes research completed with cognitively healthy adults, people living with dementia from various etiologies, as well as those with Alzheimer's disease, aphasia, traumatic brain injury, multiple sclerosis, Parkinson's disease, and HIV/ AIDS. Details about study subjects and their memory loss conditions are provided when available. Icons are included with each summary to identify the aspect of SR that the research explored. We expect that as research continues, with reliable evidence for a wider range of people with memory loss conditions, the SR procedure will become more refined and, therefore, will be even more effective.

(1913 [1885]) Ebbinghaus

Ebbinghaus used himself as the only subject in studying the effect of retention intervals on memory. He presented himself with a series of 6–8 novel nonsense syllables for memorization. Ebbinghaus then tested himself for free recall (i.e., recall of information in any order when not prompted or cued). To ensure free recall was not accidental, he set two consecutive error-free recalls as mastery criterion. He conducted follow-up testing from several minutes post memorization up to 31 days. Results showed that with each test Ebbinghaus required fewer trials to re-learn the information. This study laid the foundation for modern-day SR.

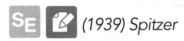 (1939) Spitzer

3,605 healthy sixth grade students in the state of Iowa were examined to study the effects of recall on retention of novel information. Subjects were divided into nine groups to manipulate test time and number of identical tests. These groups practiced recalling information over expanding periods of time using a single test condition. Regular classroom teachers presented materials for the students to read, and a 25-question, multiple-choice test was then used to assess knowledge. Results concluded that expanded practice retrievals can improve learning ability and retention.

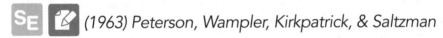 (1963) Peterson, Wampler, Kirkpatrick, & Saltzman

Thirty healthy adults participated in three experiments to determine the effect of practicing recall over progressively longer retention intervals. Pairs of words and numbers were spaced, and the spacing interval was slowly increased. Results concluded that practicing recall of information over longer time intervals increases the effectiveness of retention.

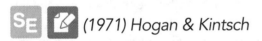 (1971) Hogan & Kintsch

Sixty-four healthy college students participated in a study testing the recognition (identifying words that were recently seen) and recall (accurately stating a specific list of words) of a 40-word list under two different conditions. In the first condition, subjects participated in one study trial followed by three recognition and recall tests, and in the second condition, subjects participated in three study trials followed by one recognition and recall test. All subjects participated in a recall and recognition test 48 hours later. Results showed that the condition with more study trials resulted in better recognition, but the condition with more recall and recognition tests facilitated better recall. A second study was also conducted with two conditions. In the first condition, subjects participated in four study trials followed by three recall tests, and in the second condition, subjects participated in one study trial followed by three recall tests. Results showed that long-term retention was better in the four study trials when measured by recognition, but better in the one study trial when measured by free recall.

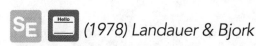 (1977) Glenberg

Four experiments were conducted with healthy adults to determine the influences of different types of recall practice techniques on the spacing effect in free recall tests (participants study a list of words and then are asked to recall the items in any order). The spacing or distance between repetitions is referred to as *lag*. Results found that the lag effect (improved recall for long lags versus short lags) was more robust when the subjects used an organizational strategy to learn, such as learning words by associating groups of items on the list. The study also found that the use of a cue word to direct retrieval produced a relationship between the cue word and what should be recalled. Results additionally found that in the absence of a cue, word retrieval can be directed with instructions.

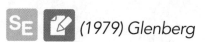 (1978) Landauer & Bjork

468 healthy adults studied pairs of items on a deck of cards, such as first names with last names, and then took three or four cued recall tests in a continuous paired-associates task, which involves the pairing of two words (a stimulus and a response). For example, words such as *dog* (stimulus) and *notebook* (response) may be paired, and when the learner is prompted with the stimulus, he or she provides the appropriate response word. Expanding and equally spaced conditions for recall and retention were created with a varied number of trials between study and test. Results showed that the expanding retrieval condition produced approximately a 10% advantage over the equally spaced practice.

SE ✍ (1979) Glenberg

Sixty-four healthy college students participated in three experiments to illustrate interactions between stored information and retrieval cues based on contextual information. Each experiment had unique conditions in which the subjects were asked to memorize word pairs or lists. In the third experiment, different study environments were provided. Following each experiment, subjects were tested for recall. Results showed that cued recall is high and unaffected by the massed practice and distributed practice variable, and in free recall retrieval is controlled by the contextual components available on the test. Additionally, variability in study environments does not affect recall on the test. Finally, the researchers suggest that under the right conditions, there may be no limit to the improvement in performance that can be achieved by increasing the space between practice intervals for free recall.

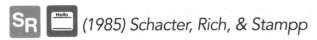 *(1985) Schacter, Rich, & Stampp*

Four subjects with memory loss resulting from various medical diagnoses were taught faces with 1–8 associated characteristics using SR. Two sessions separated with a half-hour break were given twice a week for 8 weeks. Results showed that SR assisted subjects with learning new information. Additionally, the study indicated that the technique encouraged "learning to learn" because two of the four subjects learned to use SR without cues from the researchers.

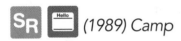 *(1989) Camp*

One subject with Alzheimer's disease was trained with SR to recall the name of a person from one photograph. Intervals were filled with conversation or games to prevent rehearsal of the learned name. Following training, the subject demonstrated the ability to retain face–name association over a 1-week interval. This procedure was replicated with two men (ages 67 and 68, respectively) with Alzheimer's disease who were trained to recall names of staff members who worked where they lived. SR was provided once a week for 30 minutes across a 3-week period. During time intervals, the subjects engaged in conversation, looked at books, or played games. Following training, both subjects were able to recall face–name associations. This study concluded that the use of SR might be practical for those with dementia.

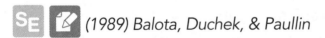 *(1989) Balota, Duchek, & Paullin*

Sixty healthy young and older adults were taught pairs of words that were presented once and then twice. They were tested in a continuous cued-recall pattern (consecutive practice rather than spaced) after either a short- or long-retention interval. Age-related differences in the lag effect and its relation to retention intervals were studied, and results showed that older adults performed lower than younger adults in recall performance. Older adults encoded less contextual information that was available and across time had slower rates of contextual fluctuation (changes in one's mental context over time).

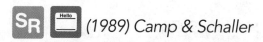 ### (1989) Camp & Schaller

One subject with memory loss was trained to learn the name of a caregiver using SR during two practice sessions. At a 6-month follow-up testing, the subject demonstrated retention of the trained information.

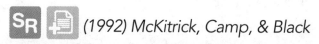 ### (1992) McKitrick, Camp, & Black

Four subjects with Alzheimer's disease were trained using SR to recall a future task and then the task requirements were adjusted after retention. The subjects were trained to remember to give the researcher a specific color coupon at the beginning of the next session. Following a 1-week maintenance interval, the subjects were then trained to remember a new coupon color. All subjects were able to learn the first task and then make adjustments to learn the second task.

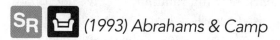 ### (1993) Abrahams & Camp

Two subjects with dementia and anomia were trained to name target objects from the Boston Naming Test (Kaplan, Goodglass, & Weintrab, 1983). SR training utilized black and white line drawings, and generalization was successfully measured by having the subjects name colored drawings and then the concrete objects. One subject participated in a 2-week maintenance session due to a sudden decline in cognitive status. Her Mini-Mental State Evaluation (Folstein, Folstein, & McHugh, 1975) score had declined, but she was able to name one of two objects from her training.

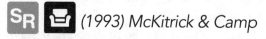 ### (1993) McKitrick & Camp

One subject with dementia was trained during 10 weekly sessions to relearn forgotten names of familiar objects from the Boston Naming Test (Kaplan, Goodglass, & Weintrab, 1983). The caregiver facilitated a SR practice using pictures or objects. After training, the subject learned all items and produced their names with much greater consistency. The caregiver reported that she was pleased with both the results of the training and the ease of using SR formally and informally.

(1993) Stevens, O'Hanlon, & Camp

One subject with Alzheimer's disease was trained using SR to use an external memory aid (a calendar) to perform tasks (which changed weekly) during weekly sessions. At the conclusion of the study, the person was able to remember to check the calendar.

   (1994) Wilson, Baddeley, Evans, & Shiel

Six studies were conducted to examine if new information can be taught to neurologically impaired adults with severe memory impairment and to observe if errorless learning is more beneficial than errorful learning. In the first study, 16 adults with amnesia were taught two lists of words under the errorless or errorful learning condition and then compared to two control groups. Results showed that errorless learning was more effective at helping people to learn new information. The five additional studies were case studies that used errorless learning to teach subjects with severe memory impairment to learn names of objects and people, to program memory aids, to remember items, and to learn items of general knowledge. Each case study found that errorless learning is superior to errorful learning.

  (1995) Bird, Alexopoulos, & Adamowicz

Five subjects with dementia were taught the association between a cue and a behavior, or a cue and information affecting the behavior, to decrease targeted problem behaviors (obsessive demands, inappropriate urination, aggressive behaviors, and persistent shouting). SR was used alone or with fading cues over one to three sessions that were 1–3 hours in length. Four of the five subjects showed a decrease in problem behaviors following training.

  (1996) Bird & Kinsella

Twenty-four subjects with dementia were trained to recall a motor task. SR and a written word cue were used to initiate performance of motor tasks, such as opening a box or reading a book. At the conclusion of the study, it was found that retrieval combined with motor performance increased the probability of task performance at final recall.

(1996) Hayden & Camp

Two men (ages 63 and 79, respectively) with dementia associated with Parkinson's disease were taught a verbal task, a motor task, or a motor–verbal task to explore the efficacy of using SR for motor or verbal learning with this population. Results showed that at follow-up testing, the first subject was able to recall one of two verbal tasks, and the second subject was able to recall the motor task and the motor–verbal task. These results indicated that patterns of memory and cognitive deficits in individuals with Parkinson's disease vary from person to person, and SR is a promising intervention to address these concerns. Additionally, the authors state that further research is needed on cognitive interventions for dementia in Parkinson's disease.

  (1997) Carruth

Seven subjects with memory loss were examined to determine the effects of singing the target response during SR practice to teach face–name associations. The SR procedure was slightly modified in the music condition by having the therapist sing a song once and then inviting the participant to sing along. After singing the song twice, the therapist used the remaining time to implement SR. Results indicated that music therapy combined with SR is beneficial for face–name associations in people with memory loss.

  (1997) Camp & Foss

An older man with dementia living in a care center was trained to recall a staff member's name. SR was implemented once a week for 30 minutes. At the conclusion of training, he could recall the nurse's name; however, he still referred to her as "nurse" because he felt it would not be polite to call her by her first name. Researchers encouraged the nurse to use expanding intervals to request that he use her name. After several exchanges at expanding intervals, the subject began to use the nurse's name. The authors concluded that real-world settings might play a role in the outcome of treatments more so than a controlled laboratory environment.

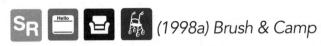 *(1998a) Brush & Camp*

Nine people with memory loss resulting from a stroke or dementia were studied to determine whether SR could be an effective intervention during speech-language therapy. SR was used to assist the participants in learning the therapist's name; one piece of information in an area important to each participant; and a compensatory technique, such as using a schedule, describing an item when unable to recall the name, or using strategies to increase vocal intensity. Results indicated that SR assisted participants in learning and using information in a functional manner, which facilitated achievement of the speech-language therapy goals.

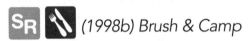 *(1998b) Brush & Camp*

One subject with memory loss and dysphagia was trained to remember and use compensatory strategies for safe swallowing. SR was combined with a visual cue card placed in front of the food tray. At the conclusion of the study, the subject required instruction only once during mealtime, and at the 8-week follow up, recall occurred 95% of the time with one reminder during mealtime.

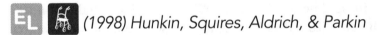 *(1998) Hunkin, Squires, Aldrich, & Parkin*

One adult with memory impairment was taught basic word processing skills using errorless learning over 30 sessions. The word processing task was broken down hierarchically. In addition, an incremental learning procedure was applied that allowed the subject to learn and practice a skill before being taught a new one. The subject showed improvement on all exercises and was able to use skills to perform the same tasks without instructions.

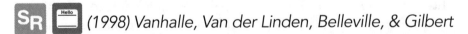 *(1998) Vanhalle, Van der Linden, Belleville, & Gilbert*

One subject with Alzheimer's disease was trained to make face–name associations using SR. The study aimed to determine if SR was more effective when favoring implicit versus explicit memory. During the implicit condition, the subject was asked to say the first name, which crossed her mind when she saw the face. In the explicit condition, the subject was asked to remember the learning context. It was explained that she had been shown the face before in the experiment, and she was then asked to recall the name of the person pictured. The subject reached criterion for the two face–name associations in the implicit condition, but failed to recall the face–name associations in the explicit condition. Results indicated that SR is beneficial when targeting implicit memory.

  (1999) Cherry & Simmons-D'Gerolamo

Six subjects with probable Alzheimer's disease were trained to recall names of objects. SR was used during three training sessions on alternate days during 1 week. Participants selected a target object from an array of items at increasingly longer retention intervals. Three subjects were given a target object orientation task in which participants responded to a sequence of three questions to solicit informal conversation about the target object prior to training. Results indicated that the orientation task had a positive effect on recall of the target object across trials and supported the concept that task-relevant orienting activities increase the strength of SR.

  (1999) Cherry, Simmons, & Camp

Four subjects with probable Alzheimer's disease were trained to recall names of everyday objects. SR was used on alternate days during 1 week. At the conclusion of the study, it was found that SR enhanced retention within and across sessions for all subjects.

  (2001) Anderson, Arens, Arens, & Coppens

Six subjects with mild to moderate dementia were provided memory tape training (repeated listening to tape-recorded information with 10 seconds in between each piece of information) or SR practice to enhance recall of personal information. Results indicated that both treatment techniques were effective forms of memory rehabilitation. However, the subjects who received SR learned the target information in less time when compared to those who received practice listening to tape recordings of information. Additionally, those who received SR demonstrated carryover.

  (2001) Bird

Two subjects with memory loss were taught to replace undesired behaviors with appropriate behaviors using SR and fading cues. Subject

1 had been engaging in violence related to delusions that someone had stolen her belongings, and subject 2 had used the restroom obsessively because he was afraid of soiling himself. External memory aids (a poster for subject 1 and an alarm for subject 2) were used to prompt recall of the appropriate behaviors. Results indicated that the use of an external memory aid paired with SR is effective in achieving clinical goals for participant-specific problems.

   (2001) Davis, Massman, & Doody

Thirty-seven subjects with probable Alzheimer's disease were divided into two conditions and participated in 1-hour weekly sessions for 5 weeks. Subjects in the first group acted as a control group by participating in unstructured conversation with the researcher, answering questions about the state of their memory, reciting overlearned material, and watching videos about general health issues. The second group participated in SR and tasks designed to enhance thinking and reasoning skills. Results showed that the second condition demonstrated significant improvement in recall of personal information, face–name recall, and performance on the Verbal Series Attention Test (Mahurin & Cooke, 1996). However, improvement did not generalize to caregiver-assessed patient quality of life or to additional neuropsychological measures of dementia severity, verbal memory, visual memory, word generation, and motor speed.

 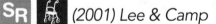 *(2001) Lee & Camp*

Two case studies were conducted to explore the effectiveness of SR when used with people who have cognitive deficits caused by HIV. The first subject was a 53-year-old male with HIV and mild dementia. He was trained to recall the name of an unknown woman in a photo. He was also trained to perform a three-step motor response as follows: pick up a card, give it to the researcher, and respond verbally. The second subject was a 64-year-old male with HIV, moderate- to severe-cognitive impairment, and blindness. He was given a photograph and told the first and last name of the person pictured. Next, he was trained to hand the researcher a coin (either a dime or a quarter). SR was provided twice a week across 2 weeks for 30 minutes, and was trained on one target skill at a time for four sessions. After two sessions for each task, the first subject was able to recall target information and demonstrated maintenance at a 2-week follow-up session. The second subject was unable to complete 30% of the training sessions due to drowsiness and apathy, but was able to recall the target name over a 2-day interval and perform all steps of the coin task over a 5-day interval. This participant was too ill to participate in the 2-week follow-up session. The authors concluded that SR appears to be a useful cognitive intervention for older adults with HIV.

  (2002) Lekeu, Wojtasik, Van der Linden, & Salmon

Two subjects were trained to use their mobile phones. SR was used to teach the subjects to consult a card posted on the back of the phone with detailed information on how to use the phone. Errorless learning was then used to help the subjects practice making calls from the phone. Training took place 1–2 days each week for 3 months. At the conclusion of the study, both subjects were able to correctly make a phone call with decreased need to consult the instruction card.

  (2003) Bourgeois, Camp, Rose, White, Malone, Carr, et al.

With the help of external memory aids, 25 subjects with dementia were taught to increase social skills, activities of daily living, and overall participation in activities. The subjects received SR and a modified cuing hierarchy to learn two personalized strategies. A cuing hierarchy involves evaluating an individual's response to every stimulus to create a hierarchy of cues based on each cue's power to elicit the desired response. Cues at the highest hierarchy provide information most likely to elicit the desired result from the participant. A modified cuing hierarchy uses the cue with the highest likelihood of eliciting the correct response from the participant first. Results showed that while both training procedures were effective, significantly more goals were attained using SR. In addition, SR goals were maintained at 1-week and 4-month follow-up sessions compared to the modified cuing hierarchy goals.

  (2003) Joltin, Camp, & McMahon

Three subjects with dementia were taught to recall the names of their family members using SR over the telephone at a minimum of three times a week for 4 weeks. Results concluded that SR could be a successful treatment modality when provided over the telephone for people with memory loss and normal hearing.

(2004) Cherry & Simmons-D'Gerolamo

Four subjects with probable Alzheimer's disease were taught to recall everyday objects from an array of objects. Two of the subjects had previously been taught using SR (approximately 2 years post training), and two who had not participated in SR training acted as controls. Six 1-hour sessions were conducted on alternate days across 2 weeks. All subjects demonstrated the positive effects of SR across sessions, as reflected in fewer errors per trial and longer retention duration across sessions. Little evidence was found to support the long-term effects of SR, but the authors asserted that future research could examine follow-up sessions for maintenance.

  (2004) Hawley & Cherry

Six subjects with probable Alzheimer's disease were taught to transfer recall of name–face association from a picture to an actual person. SR took place during six sessions across 2 weeks. Results showed a positive effect of SR for name–face recognition.

  (2004) Hochhalter, Bakke, Holub, & Overmier

Ten subjects with dementia were taught to recall one pill name with SR and one pill name with uniform retrieval training (intervals between practices are the same, not gradually increased). At the conclusion of the study, 80% of the subjects were able to recall the pill name when taught using SR, and none were able to recall the pill name taught using consecutive practice.

   (2004) Neundorfer, Camp,
Lee, Skrajner, Malone, & Carr

Ten subjects over the age of 50 with executive functioning and cognitive deficits associated with HIV/AIDS participated in 30-minute sessions twice a week across 4 weeks. SR was used to improve performance of two self-selected functional tasks using memory aids (pill organizer, calendar, timer, checklists, and cue cards). At a 2-month follow up, all participants reported that the intervention was able to help them meet their two self-selected functional goals, and the majority successfully learned and retained the correct memory strategy. The study concluded that SR paired with an external aid is a successful means to help people with HIV adhere to treatment procedures.

  (2005) Cherry & Simmons-D'Gerolamo

Ten subjects with probable Alzheimer's disease were taught to recall everyday objects from an array of objects. Five subjects had previously been taught using SR (approximately 6 months to 1 year post training), and five subjects who had not been taught using SR were included for comparison. Four of the subjects (two who had previous experience with SR and two who had not) were given a target object orientation task prior to training. Results showed that subjects with prior experience with SR had improved recall of the target information, and that the orientation task enhanced memory of the target objects.

  (2005) Fridriksson, Holland, Beeson, & Morrow

Three subjects with aphasia and moderate to severe anomia were taught 60 words of their choosing (for functional relevance) to determine usefulness of SR for individuals with aphasia. Half of the words were used for oral naming treatment and half of the words were used for writing treatment. Words used for oral training were divided between SR and a cuing hierarchy treatment. Results showed that SR was superior to a cuing hierarchy for acquisition and retention of items. The study further confirmed that SR is an effective means to improve naming of objects for individuals with aphasia.

  (2005) Hochhalter, Overmier, Gasper, Bakke, & Holub

Two studies were conducted to determine if SR is more effective than other schedules of practice. The first study compared five schedules of practice, including SR, with a verbal task. Eleven subjects with Alzheimer's disease were trained to recall pill names from a picture of the pill itself. Training was conducted four to seven times a week until long-term retention was demonstrated, or for eight sessions. At the conclusion of the study, no superior schedule of practice was identified. Two subjects demonstrated long-term retention with all five schedules of practice, while four subjects never showed long-term retention. The second study compared the same five schedules of practice using a nonverbal task replicating the procedures in the first experiment. Four subjects with dementia were trained to complete a connect-the-dots task. Results showed that three subjects demonstrated long-term retention of the nonverbal task with all five training sessions. The authors concluded that there is no evidence that SR is more likely to produce long-term retention of nonverbal information than other schedules of practice.

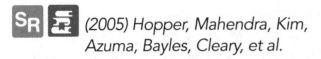 *(2005) Hopper, Mahendra, Kim, Azuma, Bayles, Cleary, et al.*

This evidence-based systematic review evaluated 15 studies to support the use of SR training for individuals with dementia. Researchers determined that the studies reviewed were positive and promising, but they identified some methodological shortcomings, indicating that the literature at the time should be interpreted with caution. This review also outlined appropriate candidates for SR, how to implement the procedure, and expected outcomes.

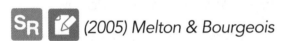 *(2005) Melton & Bourgeois*

Seven subjects with memory loss resulting from traumatic brain injury were taught to use memory aids for tasks related to prospective memory (remembering to do something in the future) and episodic memory (memory related to the time and place an event occurred) using SR over the telephone. Each subject was taught three consecutive goals for 30 minutes daily until mastery of each goal was achieved. The authors observed for goal attainment and generalization. Results showed goal attainment and generalization could be achieved in an average of five 30-minute sessions, and 94.4% of goals were maintained at 1 month post mastery with strategy execution for 77.7% of goals trained. These results indicate that using SR via the telephone is an effective means of treatment for people with traumatic brain injury.

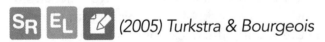 *(2005) Turkstra & Bourgeois*

This case study presents an individual with profound anterograde amnesia resulting from traumatic brain injury. The subject and caregiver identified three functional memory goals. SR, with a focus on errorless learning, was implemented over the telephone 4 days weekly for 30 minutes until mastery of each goal was achieved. Results concluded that SR with careful attention to errors is beneficial.

(2006) Balota, Duchek, Sergent-Marshall, & Roediger III

Subjects who were young adults, healthy adults, or people with Alzheimer's disease were included in three experiments comparing different schedules of retrieval practice (103, 109, and 25 subjects, respectively). The schedules included massed practice, equally spaced practice, and expanded retrieval practice, with Experiment 2 and Experiment 3 including corrective feedback. Subjects were taught to remember weakly associated word pairs from Tulving and Thomson (1973). Results showed that in Experiment 1, expanded retrieval was superior to equal-interval retrieval during acquisition, but this benefit was lost in final cued recall. In Experiments 2 and 3, there was no evidence of a difference between expanded and equal-interval conditions in final cued recall even with the addition of corrective feedback.

  (2006) Fridriksson, Morrow-Odom, Moser, Fridriksson, & Baylis

Three subjects with aphasia and anomia and two control subjects were taught to name 15 objects of their choosing using SR, errorless learning, and massed practice. No treatment items were duplicated across participants. Ten 4-hour sessions were held across 2 weeks with 5–6 fMRI scanning sessions. The study aimed to examine changes of cortical activity during training using fMRI. Results showed that two of the three subjects with aphasia benefitted from the naming treatment, and in both cases changes in cortical activity were noted.

  (2006) Morrow & Fridriksson

Three subjects with aphasia were taught to name 30 target items using SR with fixed intervals and randomized intervals to determine if strict management of SR intervals is necessary. Results concluded that neither approach appeared to be superior to the other when treating people with aphasia. However, it was noted that fewer fixed-interval SR sessions were needed and that more fixed-interval SR items were maintained during follow-up testing after treatment ended. This difference was minimal. The study suggests that a less-stringent stimulus schedule may be acceptable when used for treating people with aphasia.

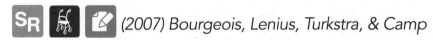 *(2007) Bourgeois, Lenius, Turkstra, & Camp*

Thirty-eight subjects with traumatic brain injury were taught three memory-related goals using SR or teaching instruction over the telephone. Each subject also had a caregiver who was willing to assist him or her and report outcomes. Subjects were divided into two groups and were paired to receive equal time over the telephone. Sessions were 30 minutes and held 4–5 days each week. Results showed that subjects in the SR group reported significantly more goal mastery than those who received teaching instruction at the end of the study and 1 month after the completion of the study. Subjects' caregivers reported similar significant differences between both groups. Significant differences or improvement in quality of life were not reported for generalized strategy use in either group. These results suggest that use of SR over the telephone is more effective than teaching instruction.

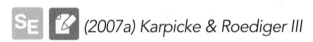 *(2007a) Karpicke & Roediger III*

Sixty healthy college students participated in two experiments examining the effects of testing on multi-trial free recall. Subjects learned lists of words across multiple study and test trials and took a final recall test 1 week after learning the words. In the first experiment, results showed that repeated testing during learning improved retention relative to repeated studying, although alternating study and test trials produced the best retention. In the second experiment, recalled items were eliminated from further studying and testing to observe how different types of practice affect retention. Results showed that repeated study of previously learned items did not benefit retention when the items were removed from further study, but repeated recall of previously recalled items enhanced retention by more than 100% relative to dropping those items from further testing. The studies concluded that repeated retrieval of information is the key to long-term retention.

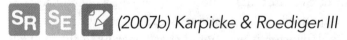 *(2007b) Karpicke & Roediger III*

Forty-eight healthy college students participated in three experiments examining the use of expanding and equally spaced retrieval practice. Experiments 1 and 2 involved teaching 52 vocabulary word pairs during five different spacing conditions with one control group. In experiment 2, subjects were given feedback about their performance. Results showed that in the presence or absence of feedback, expanding retrieval practice produced short-term benefits 10 minutes after learning, but the equally spaced retrieval practice produced better retention days later. Experiment 3 was modified by adding four more vocabulary words and by scheduling the first test to occur immediately or after a brief delay. Repeated tests were given using expanding or equally spaced retrieval practice. Results showed that expanding the interval between repeated tests had little effect on long-term retention. The authors state that the key to promoting long-term recall is to delay initial retrieval to make retrieval more difficult, as is done in equally spaced retrieval but not in expanding retrieval.

(2007) Kinsella, Ong, Storey, Wallace, & Hester

Two experiments were conducted with people with Alzheimer's disease to examine whether SR could substantially improve performance of a prospective memory task. In the first experiment, 14 subjects with mild Alzheimer's disease and 14 healthy older adult subjects were provided instructions and then given a text-reading task. Following performance of the text-reading task, participants were asked whether they could recall the task instructions. In the second experiment, 16 subjects with mild Alzheimer's disease and 16 healthy older adult subjects were taught to remember and perform a prospective memory task under two learning conditions (SR and SR with elaborated encoding). At the conclusion of the study, those with Alzheimer's disease showed a greater benefit in the combined condition of SR with elaborated encoding when compared to the baseline condition and SR alone.

(2007) Vance & Farr

Authors of this publication reviewed the use of SR when applied to those with memory impairments related to mild cognitive impairment, Alzheimer's disease, stroke, and HIV. They suggest that nurses are qualified to assist their patients with memory loss by (1) identifying the specific needs of their patients related to memory loss, (2) educating patients and their caregivers to implement SR on their own, and (3) monitoring outcomes by checking on progress as reported by patients and caregivers as well as offering feedback.

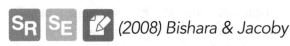 *(2008) Bishara & Jacoby*

Two experiments with 36 healthy adults were conducted to examine the effects of SR and spaced studying on controlled recollection and unconscious or automatic recall. Pairs of words were used to study memory performance in a retrieved condition compared with performance after studying word pairs by reading them. Results show SR can improve memory more effectively than spaced studying for both younger and older adults.

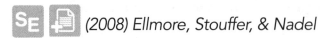 *(2008) Ellmore, Stouffer, & Nadel*

Two experiments were conducted with healthy college students to determine how much time is required for retrieval of explicit and implicit memories after retention intervals and to determine how the explicit and implicit processing times change when the associations are rehearsed after initial retrieval. The study found that the time it took to retrieve the explicit component increased when compared to baseline and decreased after spaced retrieval, but not significantly. Additionally, the implicit processing times continued to gradually decrease after retention. With continued rehearsal, the implicit processing times became significantly lower when compared to baseline. The authors concluded that different amounts of processing time might be required for retrieval of these different memory components.

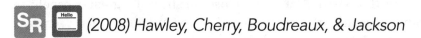 *(2008) Hawley, Cherry, Boudreaux, & Jackson*

Twelve subjects with probable Alzheimer's disease were taught to learn name–face associations using SR and uniform expanded retrieval during nine sessions on alternate days across 2 weeks. Results showed that SR had a positive effect on the proportion of correct recall trials and greater success in transferring the learned information to the live target when compared to the uniform expanded retrieval schedule.

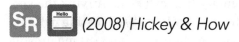 *(2008) Hickey & How*

Three subjects with dementia were taught to read nametags of staff caregivers using SR. Written cues were used during training if independent recall could not be achieved. At the conclusion of the study, one subject was unable to move beyond the cued-response stage of training, whereas the remaining two subjects were able to achieve the goal in seven and three sessions, respectively. One subject achieved post-training maintenance and generalization.

(2008) Karpicke & Roediger III

Forty-eight healthy college students learned a list of foreign language vocabulary words under four conditions to determine the effects of repeated studying and repeated testing on learning. Additionally, the researchers examined the relationship between the speed with which information is learned, the rate at which information is forgotten, and the students' assessment of their own learning. Results showed that repeated retrieval practice enhanced long-term retention, whereas repeated studying produced essentially no benefit to the student. Additionally, researchers found that the rate at which information is forgotten is not necessarily determined by the speed of learning; the type of practice involved has a greater impact. Finally, students' predictions of their own performance were uncorrelated with actual performance.

(2008) Lee, Park, Jeong, Choe, Hwang, Park, et al.

Nineteen subjects with dementia participated in 24 SR sessions to measure efficacy of SR on the cognition of people with very mild and mild Alzheimer's disease and to assess changes in neuropsychological performance after SR. All test batteries were administered in the Korean language, and all training targets were disyllabic words in the Korean language. Study outcomes showed that retention spans were significantly increased after SR in both very mild and mild Alzheimer's disease subjects. This improvement was maintained for different sets of target information. The number of words retained also significantly increased after SR for the very mild Alzheimer's disease subjects. No changes were observed in neuropsychological performance after SR.

(2008) Logan & Balota

194 healthy younger and older adults were taught low association words using SR and expanded retrieval to investigate potential age-related differences in the ability to recall words and the benefit of each method. Both groups showed a memory advantage for expanded items compared to equal interval items during the learning phase. After a 24-hour delay, older adults showed no expanded retrieval advantage, and younger

adults showed a disadvantage. Results indicate that both younger and older adults experienced substantial benefits from spaced (vs. massed) retrieval practice, no matter which form it took (expanded or equal interval practice).

  (2008) Ozgis, Rendell, & Henry

Forty healthy older adults and 30 cognitively impaired older adults were taught to improve prospective memory tasks related to daily activities using SR or a standard rehearsal condition. Results showed that both subject groups benefited from SR and that enhancement effects were substantial for the cognitively impaired older adults.

  (2008) Pavlik & Anderson

Sixty subjects under the age of 49 were taught a set of 180 Japanese/English vocabulary words under three learning conditions. The study took place over three learning sessions in 1 week, with a fourth session used for assessment. The first condition used an algorithm to determine decision criteria for increasing or decreasing spacing of when each word was presented for practice. In the second condition, the first presentation of each word was a study-only presentation of the pair, with subsequent presentations always recall or restudy trials. Finally, the third condition used six stacks of 30 pairs of flashcards during learning. Results indicated that systematically spacing the presentation of each word for practice resulted in better, faster recall of the information.

   (2008) Thivierge, Simard, Jean, & Grandmaison

Two subjects were taught telephone-related tasks during two weekly sessions across 4 weeks using SR and errorless learning. Subject 1 was trained to use his voicemail, and subject 2 was trained to manage messages from his answering machine. Results showed that SR combined with errorless learning improved performance on the trained tasks, and this performance was able to be maintained over a 5-week period.

  (2009) Bier, Macoir, Gagnon,
Van der Linden, Louveaux, & Desrosiers

This study involved one subject and explored the efficacy of formal-semantic therapy and SR to restore lost concepts. Formal-semantic therapy consisted of giving feedback related to the meaning of a word followed by a cuing technique to facilitate naming. Formal-semantic therapy with simple repetition was compared to formal-semantic therapy with SR. Sessions were twice a week for 3 weeks and consisted of training using picture-naming tasks and verbal naming of attributes. Study outcomes showed that the subject's ability to name items based on training using picture-naming tasks increased along with the subject's performance in verbally naming the specific semantic attributes of concepts. Additionally, the subject was able to maintain the improved performance over a 5-week period.

  (2009) Cherry, Hawley, Jackson, & Boudreaux

Six subjects with probable Alzheimer's disease were taught to recall name–face associations using SR. Booster sessions were given to half of the participants at 6, 12, and 18 weeks to assist in long-term retention. Results indicated that there was a benefit to providing the booster sessions at retest and demonstrated that SR supported recall of a name–face association over a 6-month interval.

 (2009) Gonzalez Rothi, Fuller, Leon, Kendall, Moore, Wu, et al.

Six subjects with Alzheimer's disease were taught with errorless learning and provided an acetyl cholinesterase inhibitor to examine if confrontation-naming ability (stating the name of an object when presented with the object or a picture of the object) would improve. Subjects practiced producing the target word during 60-minute sessions four times a week for 5–9 weeks. Results showed significant improvements in verbal confrontation naming of trained items for three subjects. The authors suggest further treatment studies examining the use of language treatment in combination with acetyl cholinesterase inhibitor.

   (2009) Neely, Vikstrom, & Josephsson

This study involved 30 subjects with dementia and their spouses (60 subjects total) and examined the effectiveness of a collaborative memory intervention. The three conditions included a collaborative condition that involved the participating caregiver, a condition where the same training was provided without the participating caregiver, and a control group that did not receive training. SR was used in sessions once per week across 8 weeks to teach face–name recall along with hierarchical cuing, which was also used to teach a table-setting activity. Results showed that the collaborative condition resulted in tasks becoming more equally shared between the person with dementia and his or her spouse, with the person with dementia demonstrating increased participation in tasks and recall of information when comparing pre-test with post-test. Additionally, in the collaborative condition, the spouse with dementia improved his or her individually assessed episodic memory performance compared to the remaining two conditions. Finally, training had no effects on episodic memory, perceived burden, or depressive symptoms for the caregivers, but the results of the training did imply that the active participation of the caregiver matters in cognitive dementia rehabilitation.

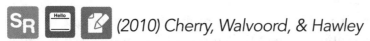 *(2010) Cherry, Walvoord, & Hawley*

Four subjects with probable Alzheimer's disease were taught to recall name–face–occupation association and to transfer the information to the live person used in training photos. For instance, when the person saw the face of a nurse, the goal was to recall the person's name and that he or she was a nurse. SR was implemented during six sessions across 2 weeks. Results showed the positive effects of SR on memory for name–face–occupation recall, with occupation being recalled more than the person's name. Modest evidence was reported for transfer of the learned information to the actual person.

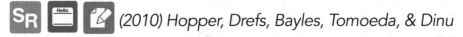 *(2010) Hopper, Drefs, Bayles, Tomoeda, & Dinu*

This study examined 32 subjects with dementia to determine the effects of SR on the learning of new and previously known associations. SR was implemented in either a related condition where time intervals between practices were filled with activities related to the information being learned, or an unrelated condition where time intervals between practices were filled with activities not related to the information being learned. Results showed that previously known associations were learned significantly faster than new associations, with retention lasting for variable amounts of time up to 6 weeks. Furthermore, the activities used during the time intervals between practices did not speed the learning or lengthen the time of retention.

(2010) Lin, Huang, Su, Watson, Tsai, & Wu

Eighty-five subjects with dementia were studied to investigate the effectiveness of SR and Montessori-based activities in decreasing eating difficulty. Subjects were organized under an SR condition, Montessori-based condition, or control condition and were provided three 30–40 minute sessions per week across 8 weeks. Results showed that assisted feeding scores for the SR and Montessori-based conditions were significantly lower than that of the control group; however, subjects in the Montessori-based condition needed more physical and verbal assistance during mealtimes. Finally, the nutritional status after intervention improved more significantly for subjects in the SR condition than for those in the control group.

  (2010) Sumowski, Chiaravalloti, & DeLuca

Thirty-two subjects with multiple sclerosis were matched to 16 healthy control subjects and were taught 48 low-associated word pairs using three conditions—mass practice, spaced study, and spaced testing. The authors observed which procedure was more efficient at improving memory performance of subjects with multiple sclerosis. At the conclusion of the study, both groups had a high rate of success with the spaced testing condition, indicating that retrieval practice is more effective at improving memory when compared to restudy for people with neurologically-based memory impairment.

  (2010) Sumowski, Wood, Chiaravalloti, Wylie, Lengenfelder, & DeLuca

Fourteen subjects with traumatic brain injury were matched to 14 healthy control subjects and were taught 48 low-associated word pairs using mass practice, spaced study, and retrieval practice. The authors used the three conditions to observe which procedure is more efficient at improving memory performance of subjects with traumatic brain injury. At the conclusion of the study, both groups greatly benefited from the retrieval practice condition when compared to mass practice and spaced study. Results indicated that retrieval practice improves memory for people with traumatic brain injury even when other memory learning strategies are less effective.

(2010) Vance, Struzick, & Farr

Authors of this publication reviewed the use of SR with various populations and concluded that the SR strategy is a practical way for social workers to help clients compensate for memory loss related to activities of daily living. They suggest that during SR time intervals, social workers can talk with clients about other issues. They first recommend that social workers become familiar with the mechanisms that account for SR's success prior to implementation. Next, social workers should (1) identify clients who are already at risk of experiencing memory problems and who can benefit from SR, (2) educate clients and their caregivers on implementing SR on their own, and (3) communicate with clients and caregivers during and after SR sessions to assess effectiveness and offer feedback.

  (2011) Haslam, Hodder, & Yates

Three experiments were conducted comparing the effectiveness of SR and errorless learning when working with people with dementia and traumatic brain injury. Sixty healthy control subjects, 30 subjects with traumatic brain injury, and 15 subjects with dementia were taught to recall face–name associations. Both SR and errorless learning resulted in improved accuracy in completing the trained task across all subjects, but SR was significantly better when compared to errorless learning.

  (2011) Karpicke & Bauernschmidt

Ninety-six healthy college students participated in a study to determine the relationship between spacing schedules and patterns of response times and the relationship between patterns of response times and final recall. Subjects learned 100 Swahili/English word pairs during 12 spacing conditions separated into four groups: short spacing, medium spacing, long spacing, and a no spacing control condition. Subjects then practiced recalling the items on three repeated tests that were distributed according to one of several spacing schedules determined by a computer program. Results showed that increasing the spacing of repeated tests produced large effects on long-term retention when compared to repeated retrieval with no spacing between tests. However, there was no evidence that one spacing schedule was superior to another. The authors concluded that repeated SR is very effective with retention, but that the schedule of repeated tests has no impact on outcomes.

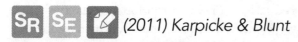 *(2011) Karpicke & Blunt*

Eighty healthy college students participated in a study to examine the effectiveness of retrieval practice and elaborative studying with concept mapping in two experiments. In the first experiment, students studied a science text across four conditions that modified the number of study periods allowed in one session, with the last condition allowing for the creation of a concept map. The second experiment replicated the first experiment, but extended it by changing the structure of the text being studied, extending the subject pool to 120 healthy college students, and assessing long-term retention with two different final test formats. Results show that practicing retrieval produces more meaningful learning than elaborative studying with concept mapping.

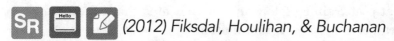 *(2012) Fiksdal, Houlihan, & Buchanan*

One subject with dementia was taught to recall names and jobs of family members that he would be seeing at an upcoming family reunion with memory priming during 3–5 weekly sessions over 3–5 weeks. The subject engaged in a 5-minute conversation about preferred topics that he identified, and then two questions were presented every 2 minutes. SR was then used to strengthen and maintain the information learned through memory priming. Results indicated that memory priming followed by SR enhances the recall of meaningful conversational information and has positive effects on helping people with dementia relearn forgotten information.

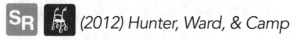 *(2012) Hunter, Ward, & Camp*

Six subjects with dementia as a result of Alzheimer's disease or vascular dementia living in a care facility in Australia were taught to resolve problem behavior identified by the care facility staff. Subjects participated in between two to nine SR sessions that lasted between 20–30 minutes over a 3-week period on consecutive days. The study investigated how SR can be transferred to staff in an aged care facility once it has been implemented with residents with dementia, with the additional goal of determining the potential barriers and facilitators to successfully transferring this strategy to staff. Additionally, the efficacy of SR in training more than one functional goal was examined. The frequency and severity of problem behaviors, as well as the distress and disturbance these behaviors caused, were recorded at baseline, post-intervention, and 3-week follow up. Results showed reductions in each area for four participants, including where two goals were trained simultaneously. The care facility staff reported that time pressure, staff turnover, and forgetting to use the SR intervention can be potential barriers to consistent implementation of the SR method. Researchers concluded that SR could be used successfully in aged care facilities to train either one or two goals.

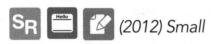 *(2012) Small*

Eight subjects with dementia were taught to remember face–name associations, object–word associations, and current events. Three SR training conditions were used to target semantic memory, prospective memory, and episodic memory during 12 sessions across 6 weeks, with two 2-hour sessions each week. Results showed gains by all participants across all conditions at post-training follow up and indicated that SR can be used to teach recall of new episodic information.

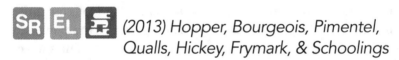 *(2013) Hopper, Bourgeois, Pimentel, Qualls, Hickey, Frymark, & Schoolings*

This evidence-based systematic review evaluated 43 studies to determine the current state of research evidence related to cognitive interventions for those with Alzheimer's disease or dementia. The most common cognitive intervention techniques analyzed were SR, errorless learning, vanishing cues, and verbal instruction or cuing. The researchers concluded that treatment outcomes showed positive effects supporting the use of cognitive interventions for individuals with dementia. However, results should be interpreted with caution because of study limitations.

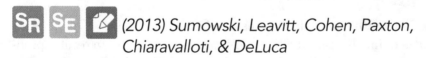 *(2013) Sumowski, Leavitt, Cohen, Paxton, Chiaravalloti, & DeLuca*

Twelve subjects with multiple sclerosis were taught 48 low-associated word pairs using three conditions. Massed restudy, spaced restudy, and retrieval practice were used to observe if retrieval practice improved memory after both short (30 minutes) and long (1 week) delays in memory-impaired multiple sclerosis patients. At the conclusion of the study, retrieval practice significantly improved memory when compared to the other conditions, indicating that retrieval practice is the best memory technique after both short and long delays for people with multiple sclerosis.

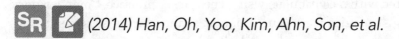 *(2013) Wu & Lin*

This study, which involved three conditions, examined the long-term effects of SR combined with Montessori-based activities on nutritional status, body mass index, and depressive symptoms (improved nutritional status has a moderating effect on depressive symptoms). SR combined with Montessori-based activities was used with 25 fixed group subjects over 24 sessions, and 38 individualized subjects received the same intervention during different sessions, with the intervention adjusted according to each participant's learning response. Finally, 27 subjects acted as a control group, receiving only routine care. Those for whom SR combined with a Montessori-based therapy was implemented showed a decrease in depressive symptoms with increased nutrition when compared to those who received routine care.

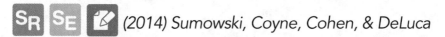 *(2014) Han, Oh, Yoo, Kim, Ahn, Son, et al.*

Ten subjects with mild cognitive impairment were studied to evaluate the feasibility and efficacy of the Ubiquitous Spaced Retrieval-based Memory Advancement and Rehabilitation Training (USMART), a self-administered program developed as an iPad app. SR was used with words derived from the USMART app. Feasibility was evaluated by checking participant satisfaction using a 5-point Likert scale, and efficacy was measured with a Korean neuropsychological assessment. Results showed that word list memory significantly increased after using the program. The authors also indicated that USMART was effective in improving memory and well tolerated by most participants.

SR SE 📝 *(2014) Sumowski, Coyne, Cohen, & DeLuca*

Ten subjects with severe traumatic brain injury were taught 48 low-associated word pairs using three conditions. Massed restudy, spaced restudy, and retrieval practice were used to observe if retrieval practice improved memory after both short (30 minutes) and long (1 week) delays. At the conclusion of the study, retrieval practice significantly improved memory when compared to the other conditions in both short and long delays. This study indicated that retrieval practice is the only effective condition for recall following long delays for people with severe traumatic brain injury.

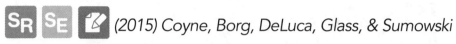 *(2015) Coyne, Borg, DeLuca, Glass, & Sumowski*

Fifteen subjects ages 8 to 16 with traumatic brain injury were taught 48 low-associated word pairs using massed restudy, spaced restudy, and retrieval practice to determine the most effective memory strategy for this population. At the conclusion of the study, retrieval practice produced a significant learning effect with better recall when compared to the other conditions. Additionally, retrieval practice was the single best learning strategy for every subject who participated in the study.

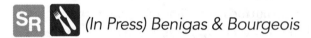 *(In Press) Benigas & Bourgeois*

Five subjects with dementia were taught to use 2–3 relevant compensatory swallowing strategies to avoid food and liquid modifications. SR was implemented with a continuous visual cue during practice. Compensatory swallowing strategies were taught one at a time during sessions lasting 30–45 minutes 5 days a week until all strategies were learned. Results, paired with social validation ratings, showed that people with dementia could learn compensatory swallowing strategies for use during oral intake.

Bibliography

Abrahams, J. P., & Camp, C. J. (1993). Maintenance and generalization of object naming training in anomia associated with degenerative dementia. *Clinical Gerontologist, 12*(3), 57–72.

Alexander, M. P., & Geschwind, N. (1984). Dementia in the elderly. In M. L. Albert (Ed.), *Clinical Neurology of Aging* (pp. 254–276). New York: Oxford University Press.

Alzheimer's Disease International. (2013). The Global Impact of Dementia 2013–2050. Retrieved from https://www.alz.co.uk/research/GlobalImpactDementia2013.pdf.

American Speech Language and Hearing Association. (2012). EBP Compendium: Summary of Systematic Review. Retrieved from http://www.asha.org/Members/ebp/compendium/reviews/Evidence-Based-Practice-Recommendations-for-Working-with-Individuals-with-Dementia--Spaced-Retr---.htm.

Americans with Disabilities Act of 1990. (1990). Pub L. No. 101–336, 104 Stat. 328. Retrieved from http://www.ada.gov/pubs/ada.htm.

Anderson, J., Arens, K., Arens, K., & Coppens, P. (2001). Spaced retrieval vs. memory tape therapy in memory rehabilitation for dementia of the Alzheimer's type. *Clinical Gerontologist, 24*(1–2), 123–139.

Baddeley, A. D. (1975). Theories of amnesia. In A. Kennedy & A. Wilkes (Eds.), *Studies in Long-Term Memory* (pp. 327–343). New York: Wiley.

Baddeley, A. D. (1992). Working memory. *Science, 255*(5044), 556–559.

Baddeley, A. D. (1999). *Essentials of Human Memory* (Vol. 1). United Kingdom: Psychology Press.

Baddeley, A. D. (2000). The episodic buffer: A new component of working memory? *Trends in Cognitive Science, 4*(11), 417–423.

Baddeley, A. D., & Hitch, G. (1974). Working memory. In G. H. Bower (Ed.), *The Psychology of Learning and Motivation: Advances in Research and Theory* (Vol. 8, pp. 47–89). New York: Academic Press.

Balota, D. A., Duchek, J. M., & Logan, J. M. (2007). Is expanded retrieval practice a superior form of spaced retrieval? A critical review of the extant literature. In J. S. Nairne (Ed.), *The Foundations of Remembering: Essays in Honor of Henry L. Roediger, III* (pp. 83–105). New York: Psychology Press.

Balota, D. A., Duchek, J. M., & Paullin, R. (1989). Age-related differences in the impact of spacing, lag, and retention interval. *Psychology and Aging, 4*(1), 3–9.

Balota, D. A., Duchek, J. M., Sergent-Marshall, S. D., & Roediger III, H. L. (2006). Does expanded retrieval produce benefits over equal-interval spacing?: Explorations of spacing effects in healthy aging and early stage Alzheimer's disease. *Psychology and Aging, 21*(1), 19.

Benigas, J. E. (2013). *Using spaced retrieval with external aids to improve use of compensatory strategies during eating for persons with dementia* (doctoral dissertation). Retrieved from https://etd.ohiolink.edu/!etd.send_file?accession=os u1373826803&disposition=inline.

Benigas, J. E., & Bourgeois, M. S. (in press). Using spaced retrieval with external aids to improve use of compensatory strategies during eating for persons with dementia. *American Journal of Speech Language Pathology.*

Bier, N., Macoir, J., Gagnon, L., Van der Linden, M., Louveaux, S., & Desrosiers, J. (2009). Known, lost, and recovered: Efficacy of formal-semantic therapy and spaced retrieval method in a case of semantic dementia. *Aphasiology, 23*(2), 210–235.

Bird, M. (2001). Behavioural difficulties and cued recall of adaptive behaviour in dementia: Experimental and clinical evidence. *Neuropsychological Rehabilitation, 11*(3–4), 357–375.

Bird, M., Alexopoulos, P., & Adamowicz, J. (1995). Success and failure in five case studies: Use of cued recall to ameliorate behaviour problems in senile dementia. *International Journal of Geriatric Psychiatry, 10*(4), 305–311.

Bird, M., & Kinsella, G. (1996). Long-term cued recall of tasks in senile dementia. *Psychology and Aging, 11*(1), 45.

Bishara, A. J., & Jacoby, L. L. (2008). Aging, spaced retrieval, and inflexible memory performance. *Psychonomic Bulletin & Review, 15*(1), 52–57.

Bjork, R. A. (1988). Retrieval practice and the maintenance of knowledge. In M. M. Gruneberg, P. E. Morris, & R. N. Sykes (Eds.), *Practical Aspects of Memory II* (pp. 396–401). London: Wiley.

Bourgeois, M. S. (1990). Enhancing conversation skills in residents with Alzheimer's disease using a prosthetic memory aid. *Journal of Applied Behavior Analysis, 23,* 29–42.

Bourgeois, M. S. (1991). Communication treatment for adults with dementia. *Journal of Speech, Language, and Hearing Research, 34*(4), 831–844.

Bourgeois, M. S. (1992a). *Enhancing the Conversations of Memory-Impaired Persons: A Memory Aid Workbook.* Gaylord, MI: Northern Speech Services, Inc.

Bourgeois, M. S. (1992b). Evaluating memory wallets in conversations with persons with dementia. *Journal of Speech and Hearing Research, 35,* 1344–1357.

Bourgeois, M. S. (1993). Effects of memory aids on the didactic conversations of individuals with dementia. *Journal of Applied Behavior Analysis, 26,* 77–87.

Bourgeois, M. S. (2013). *Memory and Communication Aids for People with Dementia.* Baltimore: Health Professions Press.

Bourgeois, M. S., Camp, C., Rose, M., White, B., Malone, M., Carr, J., et al. (2003). A comparison of training strategies to enhance use of external aids by persons with dementia. *Journal of Communication Disorders, 36*(5), 361–378.

Bourgeois, M. S., & Hickey, E. M. (2009). *Dementia: From Diagnosis to Management—A Functional Approach.* New York: Psychological Press.

Bourgeois, M. S., Lenius, K., Turkstra, L., & Camp, C. (2007). The effects of cognitive teletherapy on reported everyday memory behaviours of persons with chronic traumatic brain injury. *Brain Injury, 21*(12), 1245–1257.

Bourgeois, M. S., & Mason, L. A. (1996). Memory wallet intervention in adult day care setting. *Behavior Interventions: Theory and Practice in Residential and Community-Based Clinical Programs, 11,* 3–18.

Brush, J. A., Calkins, M. P., Bruce, C., & Sanford, J. A. (2012). *Environmental & Communication Assessment Toolkit for Dementia Care.* Baltimore: Health Professions Press

Brush, J., & Camp, C. (1998a). Using spaced retrieval training as an intervention during speech-language therapy. *Clinical Gerontologist, 19*(1), 51–64.

Brush, J., & Camp, C. (1998b). Spaced retrieval during dysphagia therapy: A case study. *Clinical Gerontologist, 19*(2), 77–99.

Brush, J. A., & Camp, C. J. (1998c). *A Therapy Technique for Improving Memory: Spaced Retrieval.* Menorah Park Center for Senior Living.

Brush, J., Camp, C., Bohach, S., & Gertsberg, N. (2015). Creating supportive wayfinding for persons with dementia. *Canadian Nursing Home, 26*(1), 4–11.

Brush, J. A., Meehan, R. A., & Calkins, M. (2002). Using the environment to improve intake for people with dementia. *Alzheimer's Care Quarterly, 3*(4), 330–338.

Calkins, M. (2002). Environments that make a difference. *Alzheimer's Care Quarterly, 3*(1), v–vii.

Camp, C. J. (1989). Facilitation of new learning in Alzheimer's disease. In G. Gilmore, P. Whitehouse, & M. Wykle (Eds.), *Memory and Dementia: Research, Theory, and Practice* (pp. 212–225). New York: Springer Publishing Company.

Camp, C. J., & Foss, J. W. (1997). Designing ecologically valid memory interventions for persons with dementia. In D. G Payne & F. G. Conrad (Eds.), *Intersections in Basic and Applied Memory Research* (pp. 311–325). Mahwah, NJ: Erlbaum.

Camp, C. J., Foss, J. W., O'Hanlon, A. M., & Stevens, A. B. (1996). Memory interventions for persons with dementia. *Applied Cognitive Psychology, 10*(3), 193–210.

Camp, C. J., & Schaller, J. R. (1989). Epilogue: Spaced retrieval memory training in an adult day care center. *Educational Gerontology: An International Quarterly, 15*(6), 641–648.

Camp, C. J., & Stevens, A. B. (1990). Spaced retrieval: A memory intervention for dementia of the Alzheimer's type. *Clinical Gerontologist: The Journal of Aging and Mental Health, 10*(1), 58–61.

Carpman, J., & Grant, M. (2001). *Design that Cares: Planning Health Facilities for Patients and Visitors.* San Francisco: Jossey-Bass, Inc.

Carruth, E. K. (1997). The effects of singing and the spaced retrieval technique on improving face-name recognition in nursing home residents with memory loss. *Journal of Music Therapy, 34*(3), 165–186.

Cherry, K. E., Hawley, K. S., Jackson, E. M., & Boudreaux, E. O. (2009). Booster sessions enhance the long-term effectiveness of spaced retrieval in older adults with probable Alzheimer's disease. *Behavior Modification, 33*(3), 295–313.

Cherry, K. E., & Simmons-D'Gerolamo, S. S. (1999). Effects of a target object orientation task on recall in older adults with probable Alzheimer's disease. *Clinical Gerontologist, 20*(4), 39–63.

Cherry, K. E., & Simmons-D'Gerolamo, S. S. (2004). Long-term effectiveness of spaced-retrieval memory training for older adults with probable Alzheimer's disease. *Experimental Aging Research, 31*(3), 261–289.

Cherry, K. E., & Simmons-D'Gerolamo, S. S. (2005). Long-term effectiveness of spaced retrieval memory training for older adults with probable Alzheimer's disease. *Experimental Aging Research, 31*(3), 261–289.

Cherry, K. E., Simmons, S. S., & Camp, C. J. (1999). Spaced retrieval enhances memory in older adults with probable Alzheimer's disease. *Journal of Clinical Geropsychology, 5*(3), 159–175.

Cherry, K. E., Walvoord, A. A., & Hawley, K. S. (2010). Spaced retrieval enhances memory for a name-face-occupation association in older adults with probable Alzheimer's disease. *The Journal of Genetic Psychology, 171*(2), 168–181.

Cohen, U., & Weisman, G. D. (1991). *Holding on to Home: Designing Environments for People with Dementia.* Baltimore: Johns Hopkins University Press.

Collins, A. M., & Loftus, R. S. (1975). A spreading activation theory of semantic processing. *Psychological Review, 82*, 407–428.

Coyne, J. H., Borg, J. M., DeLuca, J., Glass, L., & Sumowski, J. F. (2015). Retrieval practice as an effective memory strategy in children and adolescents with traumatic brain injury. *Archives of Physical Medicine and Rehabilitation, 96*(4), 742–745.

Davis, R. N., Massman, P. J., & Doody, R. S. (2001). Cognitive intervention in Alzheimer disease: a randomized placebo-controlled study. *Alzheimer Disease & Associated Disorders, 15*(1), 1–9.

Dementia Services Development Centre. (2010). *10 Helpful Hints for Dementia Design at Home*. Sydney: Hammond Press.

Ebbinghaus, H. (1913). *Memory: A Contribution to Experimental Psychology*. New York: Teachers College, Columbia University (original work published 1885).

Elliot, E. (2012). *Montessori Methods for Dementia*. Oakville, Ontario: DementiAbility Enterprises, Inc.

Ellmore, T. M., Stouffer, K., & Nadel, L. (2008). Divergence of explicit and implicit processing speed during associative memory retrieval. *Brain Research, 1229*, 155–166.

Everitt, D. E., Fields, D. R., Soumerai, S. S., & Avorn, J. (1991). Resident behavior and staff distress in the nursing home. *Journal of the American Geriatrics Society, 39*(8), 792–798.

Fiksdal, B. L., Houlihan, D., & Buchanan, J. A. (2012). Improving recall in a person with dementia: Investigating the effectiveness of memory priming and spaced retrieval in an older adult with dementia. *Clinical Case Studies, 11*(5), 393–405.

Folstein, M. F., Folstein, S. E., & McHugh, P. R. (1975). Mini-mental state: A practical method for grading the cognitive state of patients for the clinician. *Journal of Psychiatric Research, 12*(3), 189–198.

Fridriksson, J., Holland, A., Beeson, P., & Morrow, L. (2005). Spaced retrieval treatment of anomia. *Aphasiology, 19*(2), 99–109.

Fridriksson, J., Morrow-Odom, L., Moser, D., Fridriksson, A., & Baylis, G. (2006). Neural recruitment associated with anomia treatment in aphasia. *Neuroimage, 32*(3), 1403–1412.

Gilmore, G. C., & Whitehouse, P. J. (1995). Contrast sensitivity in Alzheimer's disease: A 1-year longitudinal analysis. *Optometry & Vision Science, 72*(2), 83–91.

Glenberg, A. M. (1977). Influences of retrieval processes on the spacing effect in free recall. *Journal of Experimental Psychology: Human Learning and Memory, 3*, 282–294.

Glenberg, A. M. (1979). Component-levels theory of the effects of spacing of repetitions on recall and recognition. *Memory & Cognition, 7*(2), 95–112.

Gonzalez Rothi, L. J., Fuller, R., Leon, S. A., Kendall, D., Moore, A., Wu, S. S., et al. (2009). Errorless practice as a possible adjuvant to donepezil in Alzheimer's disease. *Journal of the International Neuropsychological Society, 15*(02), 311–322.

Gottesman, L. E. (1965). Resocialization of the geriatric mental patient. *American Journal of Public Health, 55*, 1964–1970.

Han, J. W., Oh, K., Yoo, S., Kim, E., Ahn, K. H., Son, Y. J., et al. (2014). Development of the ubiquitous spaced retrieval-based memory advancement and rehabilitation training program. *Psychiatry Investigation, 11*(1), 52–58.

Hanley, I. G. (1981). The use of signposts and active training to modify ward disorientation in elderly patients. *Journal of Behavior Therapy and Experimental Psychiatry, 12*(3), 241–247.

Hanley, I. G., & Lusty, K. (1984). Memory aids in reality orientation: A single case study design. *Behavior Research Therapy, 22*, 702–712.

Hartley, J. (1994). Designing instructional text for older readers: A literature review. *British Journal of Educational Technology, 25*(3), 172–188.

Haslam, C., Hodder, K. I., & Yates, P. J. (2011). Errorless learning and spaced retrieval: How do these methods fare in healthy and clinical populations? *Journal of Clinical and Experimental Neuropsychology, 33*(4), 432–447.

Hawley, K. S., & Cherry, K. E. (2004). Spaced retrieval effects on name-face recognition in older adults with probable Alzheimer's disease. *Behavior Modification, 28*(2), 276–296.

Hawley, K. S., Cherry, K. E., Boudreaux, E. O., & Jackson, E. M. (2008). A comparison of adjusted spaced retrieval versus a uniform expanded retrieval schedule for learning a name-face association in older adults with probable Alzheimer's disease. *Journal of Clinical and Experimental Neuropsychology, 30*(6), 639–649.

Hayden, C. M., & Camp, C. J. (1996). Spaced retrieval: A memory intervention for dementia in Parkinson's disease. *Clinical Gerontologist, 16*(2), 80–82.

Hickey, E., & How, S. (Eds.) (2008). Proceedings from Clinical Aphasiology Conference 2008. *Spaced Retrieval Training for Persons with Dementia: Maintenance and Generalization*, Jackson Hole, WY.

Hochhalter, A. K., Bakke, B. L., Holub, R. J., & Overmier, J. B. (2004). Adjusted spaced retrieval training: A demonstration and initial test of why it is effective. *Clinical Gerontologist, 27*(1–2), 159–168.

Hochhalter, A. K., Overmier, J. B., Gasper, S. M., Bakke, B. L., & Holub, R. J. (2005). A comparison of spaced retrieval to other schedules of practice for people with dementia. *Experimental Aging Research, 31*(2), 101–118.

Hogan, R. M., & Kintsch, W. (1971). Differential effects of study and test trials on long-term recognition and recall. *Journal of Verbal Learning and Verbal Behavior, 10*(5), 562–567.

Holland, A. C., & Kensinger, E. A. (2010). Emotion and autobiographical memory. *Physics of Life Reviews, 7*(1), 88–131.

Hopper, T., Bourgeois, M., Pimentel, J., Qualls, C. D., Hickey, E., Frymark, T., et al. (2013). An evidence-based systematic review on cognitive interventions for individuals with dementia. *American Journal of Speech-Language Pathology, 22*(1), 126–145.

Hopper, T., Drefs, S. J., Bayles, K. A., Tomoeda, C. K., & Dinu, I. (2010). The effects of modified spaced retrieval training on learning and retention of face-name associations by individuals with dementia. *Neuropsychological Rehabilitation, 20*(1), 81–102.

Hopper, T., Mahendra, N., Kim, E., Azuma, T., Bayles, K. A., Cleary, S. J., et al. (2005). Evidence-based practice recommendations for working with individuals with dementia: Spaced retrieval training. *Journal of Medical Speech Language Pathology, 13*(4), xxvii–xxxiv.

Huitt, W., & Hummel, J. (1997). An introduction to operant (instrumental) conditioning. *Educational Psychology Interactive*. Valdosta, GA: Valdosta State University. Retrieved from http://www.edpsycinteractive.org/topics/behsys/operant.html.

Hunkin, N. M., Squires, E. J., Aldrich, F. K., & Parkin, A. J. (1998). Errorless learning and the acquisition of word processing skills. *Neuropsychological Rehabilitation, 8*(4), 433–449.

Hunter, C. E. A., Ward, L., & Camp, C. J. (2012). Transitioning spaced retrieval training to care staff in an Australian residential aged care setting for older adults with dementia: A case study approach. *Clinical Gerontologist, 35*, 1–14.

Jokel, R., Rochon, E. A., & Anderson, N. A. (2010). Errorless learning of computer-generated words in a participant with semantic dementia. *Neuropsychological Rehabilitation, 20,* 16–41.

Joltin, A., Camp, C. J., & McMahon, C. M. (2003). Spaced retrieval over the telephone: An intervention for persons with dementia. *Clinical Psychologist, 7*(1), 50–55.

Kaplan, E., Goodglass, H., & Weintrab, S. (1983). *The Boston Naming Test.* Philadelphia: Lea & Febiger.

Karpicke, J. D., & Bauernschmidt, A. (2011). Spaced retrieval: Absolute spacing enhances learning regardless of relative spacing. *Journal of Experimental Psychology: Learning, Memory, and Cognition, 37*(5), 1250–1257.

Karpicke, J. D., & Blunt, J. R. (2011). Retrieval practice produces more learning than elaborative studying with concept mapping. *Science, 331*(6018), 772–775.

Karpicke, J. D., & Roediger III, H. L. (2007a). Repeated retrieval during learning is the key to long-term retention. *Journal of Memory and Language, 57*(2), 151–162.

Karpicke, J. D., & Roediger III, H. L. (2007b). Expanding retrieval practice promotes short-term retention, but equally spaced retrieval enhances long-term retention. *Journal of Experimental Psychology: Learning, Memory, and Cognition, 33*(4), 704.

Karpicke, J. D., & Roediger III, H. L. (2008). The critical importance of retrieval for learning. *Science, 319*(5865), 966–968.

Kinsella, G. J., Ong, B., Storey, E., Wallace, J., & Hester, R. (2007). Elaborated spaced retrieval and prospective memory in mild Alzheimer's disease. *Neuropsychological Rehabilitation, 17*(6), 688–706.

Koss, E., & Gilmore, G. C. (1998). Environmental interventions and functional ability of AD patients. In B. Vellas, J. Filten, & G. Frisoni (Eds.), *Research and practice in Alzheimer's Disease* (pp. 185–191). Paris/New York: Serdi/Springer.

Landauer, T. K., & Bjork, R. A. (1978). Optimum rehearsal patterns and name learning. In M. M. Gruneberg, P. E. Morris, & R. N. Sykes (Eds.), *Practical Aspects of Memory* (pp. 625–632). London: Academic Press.

Lawton, M. P., Fulcomer, M., & Kleban, M. H. (1984). Architecture for the mentally impaired elderly. *Environment and Behavior, 16*(6), 730–757.

Lee, M., & Camp, C. J. (2001). Spaced retrieval: A memory intervention for HIV+ older adults. *Clinical Gerontologist, 22*(3/4), 131–135.

Lee, S. B., Park, C. S., Jeong, J. W., Choe, J. Y., Hwang, Y. J., Park, C. A., et al. (2008). Effects of spaced retrieval training on cognitive function in Alzheimer's disease patients. *Archives of Gerontology and Geriatrics, 49*(2), 289–293.

Lekeu, F., Wojtasik, V., Van der Linden, M., & Salmon, E. (2002). Training early Alzheimer patients to use a mobile phone. *Acta Neurologica Belgica, 102*(3), 114–121.

Lin, L. C., Huang, Y. J., Su, S. G., Watson, R., Tsai, B. W. J., & Wu, S. C. (2010). Using spaced retrieval and Montessori-based activities in improving eating ability for residents with dementia. *International Journal of Geriatric Psychiatry, 25*(10), 953–959.

Liu, L., Gauthier, L., & Gauthier, S. (1991). Spatial disorientation in persons with early senile dementia of the Alzheimer type. *American Journal of Occupational Therapy, 45*(1), 67–74.

Logan, J. M., & Balota, D. A. (2008). Expanded vs. equal interval spaced retrieval practice: Exploring different schedules of spacing and retention interval in younger and older adults. *Aging, Neuropsychology, and Cognition, 15*(3), 257–280.

Mahurin, R. K., & Cooke, N. (1996). Verbal Series Attention Test: Clinical utility in the assessment of dementia. *The Clinical Neuropsychologist, 10*(1), 43–53.

Marquardt, G., & Schmieg, P. (2009). Dementia-friendly architecture: Environments that facilitate wayfinding in nursing homes. *American Journal of Alzheimer's Disease and Other Dementias, 24*(4), 333–340.

Mateer, C., & Sohlberg, M. (1988). A paradigm shift in memory rehabilitation. In H. Whitaker (Ed.), *Neuropsychological Studies of Non-Focal Brain Injury: Dementia and Closed Head Injury* (pp. 202–225). New York: Springer-Verlag.

McClannahan, L. E., & Risley, T. R. (1974). Design of living environments for nursing home residents: Recruiting attendance at activities. *The Gerontologist, 14*, 236–240.

McGilton, K. S., O'Brien-Pallas, L. L., Darlington, G., Evans, M., Wynn, F., & Pringle, D. M. (2003). Effects of a relationship-enhancing program of care on outcomes. *Journal of Nursing Scholarship, 35*(2), 151–156.

McKitrick, L. A., & Camp, C. J. (1993). Relearning the names of things: The spaced retrieval intervention implemented by a caregiver. *Clinical Gerontologist, 14*(2), 60–62.

McKitrick, L. A., Camp, C. J., & Black, F. W. (1992). Prospective memory intervention in Alzheimer's disease. *Journal of Gerontology, 47*(5), 337–343.

Melin, L., & Gotestam, K. G. (1981).The effects of rearranging ward routines on communication and eating behaviors of psychogeriatric patients. *Journal of Applied Behavior Analysis, 14*, 47–51.

Melton, A., & Bourgeois, M. (2005). Training compensatory memory strategies via the telephone for persons with TBI. *Aphasiology, 19*(3–5), 353–364.

Morrell, R. W., & Echt, K. V. (1997). Designing written instructions for older adults: Learning to use computers. In A. D. Fisk & W. A. Rogers (Eds.), *Handbook of Human Factors and the Older Adult* (pp. 335–361). New York: Academic.

Morrow, K. L., & Fridriksson, J. (2006). Comparing fixed- and randomized-interval spaced retrieval in anomia treatment. *Journal of Communication Disorders, 39*(1), 2–11.

Neath, I., & Surprenant, A. M. (2003). *Human Memory* (2nd ed.). Belmont, CA: Wadsworth/Thompson Learning.

Neely, A., Vikstrom, S., & Josephsson, S. (2009). Collaborative memory intervention in dementia: Caregiver participation matters. *Neuropsychological Rehabilitation, 19*(5), 696–715.

Neundorfer, M. M., Camp, C. J., Lee, M. M., Skrajner, M. J., Malone, M. L., & Carr, J. R. (2004). Compensating for cognitive deficits in persons aged 50 and over with HIV/AIDS: A pilot study of a cognitive intervention. *Journal of HIV/AIDS & Social Services, 3*(1), 79–97.

Ozgis, S., Rendell, P. G., & Henry, J. D. (2008). Spaced retrieval significantly improves prospective memory performance of cognitively impaired older adults. *Gerontology, 55*(2), 229–232.

Passini, R. (2000). *Signposting Information Design.* In R. Jacobson (Ed.), *Information Design* (pp. 83–98). Cambridge, MA: MIT Press.

Passini, R., Pigot, H., Rainville, C., & Tétreault, M. H. (2000). Wayfinding in a nursing home for advanced dementia of the Alzheimer's type. *Environment and Behavior, 32*(5), 684–710.

Pavlik, P. I., & Anderson, J. R. (2008). Using a model to compute the optimal schedule of practice. *Journal of Experimental Psychology: Applied, 14*(2), 101–117.

Pavlov, I. P. (1897/1902). *The Work of the Digestive Glands.* London: Griffin.

Peterson, L. R., Wampler, R., Kirkpatrick, M., & Saltzman, D. (1963). Effect of spacing presentations on retention of a paired associate over short intervals. *Journal of Experimental Psychology, 66*(2), 206–209.

Posner, M. I., & Snyder, C. R. R. (1975). Attention and cognitive control. In R. L. Solso (Ed.), *Information Processing and Cognition: The Loyola Symposium* (pp. 55–85). Hillsdale, NJ: Erlbaum.

Reeves, I. S. K. (1985). *Color and Its Effect on Behavior Modification in Correctional / Detention Facilities*. Winter Park, FL: Green Apple Publishing.

Richard, J., & Bizzini, L. (1979). On the ontogenetic character of the Pierre Marie-Behague Test and its utilization in the study of spatial orientation by patients with senile dementia. *Acta Psychiatrica Belgica, 79*(3), 233–253.

Rosswurm, M. A., Zimmerman, S. L., Schwartz-Fulton, J., & Norman, G. A. (1986). Can we manage wandering behavior? *The Journal of Long-Term Care Administration, 14,* 5–8.

Schacter, D. L., Rich, S. A., & Stampp, M. S. (1985). Remediation of memory disorders: Experimental evaluation of the spaced-retrieval technique. *Journal of Clinical and Experimental Neuropsychology, 7*(1), 79–96.

Small, J. A. (2012). A new frontier in spaced retrieval memory training for persons with Alzheimer's disease. *Neuropsychological Rehabilitation, 22*(3), 329–361.

Smith, W. L. (May, 1988). *Behavioral Interventions in Gerontology: Management of Behavior Problems in Individuals with Alzheimer's Disease Living in the Community*. Presented at the Association for Behavior Analysis Convention. Philadelphia, PA.

Spitzer, H. F. (1939). Studies in retention. *Journal of Educational Psychology, 30*(9), 641–657.

Squire, L. (1992). Declarative and nondeclarative memory: Multiple brain systems supporting learning and memory. *Journal of Cognitive Neuroscience, 4*(3), 232–243.

Stevens, A., O'Hanlon, A., & Camp, C. (1993). The spaced retrieval method: A case study. *Clinical Gerontologist, 13*(2), 106–109.

Sumowski, J. F., Chiaravalloti, N., & DeLuca, J. (2010). Retrieval practice improves memory in multiple sclerosis: Clinical application of the testing effect. *Neuropsychology, 24*(2), 267–272.

Sumowski, J. F., Coyne, J., Cohen, A., & DeLuca, J. (2014). Retrieval practice improves memory in survivors of severe traumatic brain injury. *Archives of Physical Medicine and Rehabilitation, 95*(2), 397–400.

Sumowski, J. F., Leavitt, V. M., Cohen, A., Paxton, J., Chiaravalloti, N. D., & DeLuca, J. (2013). Retrieval practice is a robust memory aid for memory-impaired patients with MS. *Multiple Sclerosis Journal, 19*(14), 1943–1946.

Sumowski, J. F., Wood, H. G., Chiaravalloti, N., Wylie, G. R., Lengenfelder, J., & DeLuca, J. (2010). Retrieval practice: A simple strategy for improving memory after traumatic brain injury. *Journal of the International Neuropsychological Society, 16*(06), 1147–1150.

Thivierge, S., Simard, M., Jean, L., & Grandmaison, É. (2008). Errorless learning and spaced retrieval techniques to relearn instrumental activities of daily living in mild Alzheimer's disease: A case report study. *Neuropsychiatric Disease and Treatment, 4*(5), 987–999.

Tideiksaar, R. (1997). *Falling in Old Age: Prevention and Management*. New York: Springer Publishing Company.

Tulving, E., & Thomson, D. M. (1973). Encoding specificity and retrieval processes in episodic memory. *Psychological Review, 80*(5), 352.

Turkstra, L. S., & Bourgeois, M. (2005). Intervention for a modern day HM: Errorless learning of practical goals. *Journal of Medical Speech Language Pathology, 13*(3), 205–212.

U.S. Architectural and Transportation Barriers Compliance Board. (n.d.). *Americans with Disabilities Act (ADA) Accessibility Guidelines for Buildings and Facilities.* Washington, DC: U.S. Government Printing Office.

Van Wijk-Sijbesma, C. V. (2001). The best of two worlds? Methodology for participatory assessment of community water services. Delft, the Netherlands: IRC International Water and Sanitation Centre Technical Paper Series, 38.

Vance, D. E., & Farr, K. F. (2007). Spaced retrieval for enhancing memory: Implications for nursing practice and research. *Journal of Gerontological Nursing, 33*(9), 46–52.

Vance, D. E., Struzick, T., & Farr, K. (2010). Spaced retrieval technique: A cognitive tool for social workers and their clients. *Journal of Gerontological Social Work, 53*(2), 148–158.

Vanderplas, J. M., & Vanderplas, J. H. (1980). Some factors affecting legibility of printed materials for older adults. *Perceptual and Motor Skills, 50*(3), 923–932.

Vanhalle, C., Van der Linden, M., Belleville, S., & Gilbert, B. (1998). Cognitive intervention case studies: Putting names on faces: Use of a spaced retrieval strategy in a patient with dementia of the Alzheimer type. *SIG 2 Perspectives on Neurophysiology and Neurogenic Speech and Language Disorders, 8*(4), 17–21.

Wilson, B. A. (2009). *Memory Rehabilitation: Integrating Theory and Practice.* New York: Guilford Press.

Wilson, B. A., Baddeley, A., Evans, J., & Shiel, A. (1994). Errorless learning in the rehabilitation of memory impaired people. *Neuropsychological Rehabilitation, 4*(3), 307–326.

World Health Organization. (2015). Dementia (Fact sheet No. 362). Retrieved from http://www.who.int/mediacentre/factsheets/fs362/en/.

Wu, H. S., & Lin, L. C. (2013). The moderating effect of nutritional status on depressive symptoms in veteran elders with dementia: A spaced retrieval combined with Montessori-based activities. *Journal of Advanced Nursing, 69*(10), 2229–2241.

Zgola, J. M., & Bordillon, G. (2001). *Bon Appetit!: The Joy of Dining in Long-Term Care.* Baltimore: Health Professions Press.

Index

Note: *b* indicates boxes, *f* indicates figures, *p* indicates photos

Acquired immune deficiency syndrome (AIDS), 102–103, 104–105
Activities of daily living
  case examples, *see* Activities of daily living case examples
  goals of memory training, 15–16
  lead questions/responses, 23*f*
  research, 98–99, 100, 101–102, 103, 108, 112–116, 117–118
Activities of daily living case examples
  finding items, 27–28, 27*p*, 28*b*, 31*f*
  modification of procedures, 79–83, 79*p*, 81*f*, 82*f*, 84*f*
  multi-step tasks, 65–73, 65*p*, 66*f*, 67*f*, 69*f*, 71*f*–72*f*
Age-related differences, 96
AIDS/HIV research, 102–103, 104–105
Alzheimer's disease case examples
  continuous visual cues, 45–47, 45*p*, 46*b*, 46*f*
  multiple-step tasks, 65–73, 65*p*, 66*f*, 67*f*, 69*f*, 71*f*–72*f*
  see also Dementia
Alzheimer's disease research, 96–98, 100–102, 104–107, 109–111, 113–114, 117–118
  activities of daily living, 117–118
  details/information, 98, 102, 107, 109, 114
  literature reviews, 110, 118
  name recognition, 96, 100–101, 102, 110–111, 113–114
  names of objects, 104, 105–106
  remembering things to do, 97, 102, 107, 111
  see also Dementia research
Amnesia research, 106
Anger and discontinuation, 35
Anomia research, 97, 105, 107
Anterograde amnesia research, 106
Anxiety case example, 57–58, 57*p*
Aphasia research, 105, 107, 108
Assessment, *see* Progress records; Reading screening; Spaced Retrieval screening
Autobiographical memory, 7

Billing for treatment, 29
Biographical details, 7
Booster sessions, 36–37, 113–114
Brain, 3, 4, 107
Brain injury
  ease example, 54–55, 54*p*, 55*b*, 55*f*
  research, 106, 108, 115, 116, 119–120

Care team involvement
  case examples, 47, 57–58, 57*p*, 76, 77, 79, 83
  discontinuation and, 35
  implementation guidelines, 56–58, 60*b*–61*b*
  orientation/wayfinding and, 49
  see also Family care partners
Case examples
  care team involvement, 47, 57–58, 57*p*, 76, 77, 79, 83
  continuous visual cues, 45–47, 45*p*, 46*b*, 46*f*
  external memory aids, 24–25, 24*p*, 54–55, 54*p*, 55*b*, 55*f*
  finding items, 27–28, 27*p*, 28*b*, 31*f*
  implementation of Spaced Retrieval, 24–25, 24*p*
  modification of procedures, 79–83, 79*p*, 81*f*, 82*f*, 84*f*
  multiple-step tasks, 65–73, 65*p*, 66*f*, 67*f*, 69*f*, 71*f*–72*f*
  new habits over old, 73–79, 73*p*, 74*b*, 75*f*, 76*f*, 77*b*, 78*f*
  safety when standing, 85–89, 85*p*, 87*f*, 88*b*, 88*f*, 89*f*
  Spaced Retrieval screening, 18–20, 18*p*, 19*f*, 20*b*, 66, 66*f*, 67*f*, 80, 81*f*, 82, 86, 87*f*
Cell phones, *see* Phone use
Challenging behaviors, 14–15, 117–118
Child research, 94, 119–120
Choking case example, 45–47, 45*p*, 46*b*, 46*f*
  see also Swallowing
Chore list use, 55*b*